COMPACT *Research*

Herpes

Diseases and Disorders

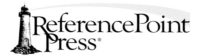

ReferencePoint Press®

San Diego, CA

Select* books in the Compact Research series include:

Current Issues

Animal Experimentation
Conflict in the Middle East
Disaster Response
DNA Evidence and
    Investigation
Drugs and Sports
Gangs
Genetic Testing
Gun Control
Immigration
Islam

National Security
Nuclear Weapons and
    Security
Obesity
Online Social
    Networking Religious
    Fundamentalism
Stem Cells
Teen Smoking
Video Games

Diseases and Disorders

ADHD
Anxiety Disorders
Bipolar Disorders
Drug Addiction
HPV
Influenza
Learning Disabilities
Mood Disorders

Obsessive-Compulsive
    Disorder
Personality Disorders
Post-Traumatic Stress
    Disorder
Self-Injury Disorder
Sexually Transmitted
    Diseases

Drugs

Antidepressants
Club Drugs
Cocaine and Crack
Hallucinogens
Heroin
Inhalants
Methamphetamine

Nicotine and Tobacco
Painkillers
Performance-Enhancing
    Drugs
Prescription Drugs
Steroids

Energy and the Environment

Biofuels
Coal Power
Deforestation
Energy Alternatives
Garbage and Recycling
Global Warming and
    Climate Change
Hydrogen Power

Nuclear Power
Oil Spills and Offshore
    Drilling
Solar Power
Toxic Waste
Wind Power
World Energy Crisis

*For a complete list of titles please visit www.referencepointpress.com.

Herpes

Charles Cozic

Diseases and Disorders

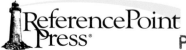

ReferencePoint
Press®

San Diego, CA

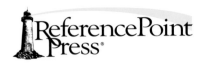

© 2011 ReferencePoint Press, Inc.
Printed in the United States

For more information, contact:
ReferencePoint Press, Inc.
PO Box 27779
San Diego, CA 92198
www.ReferencePointPress.com

LIBRARY OF CONGRESS CATALOGING-IN-PUBLICATION DATA

Cozic, Charles P., 1957–
    Herpes / by Charles Cozic.
        p. cm. — (Compact research series)
    Includes bibliographical references and index.
    ISBN-13: 978-1-60152-117-0 (hardback)
    ISBN-10: 1-60152-117-0 (hardback)
    1. Herpes genitalis. 2. Herpesvirus diseases. I. Title.
    RA644.H45C69   2011
    616.95′18—dc22
                                                    2010030634

Contents

Foreword

❝Where is the knowledge we have lost in information?❞

—T.S. Eliot, "The Rock."

As modern civilization continues to evolve, its ability to create, store, distribute, and access information expands exponentially. The explosion of information from all media continues to increase at a phenomenal rate. By 2020 some experts predict the worldwide information base will double every 73 days. While access to diverse sources of information and perspectives is paramount to any democratic society, information alone cannot help people gain knowledge and understanding. Information must be organized and presented clearly and succinctly in order to be understood. The challenge in the digital age becomes not the creation of information, but how best to sort, organize, enhance, and present information.

ReferencePoint Press developed the *Compact Research* series with this challenge of the information age in mind. More than any other subject area today, researching current issues can yield vast, diverse, and unqualified information that can be intimidating and overwhelming for even the most advanced and motivated researcher. The *Compact Research* series offers a compact, relevant, intelligent, and conveniently organized collection of information covering a variety of current topics ranging from illegal immigration and deforestation to diseases such as anorexia and meningitis.

The series focuses on three types of information: objective single-author narratives, opinion-based primary source quotations, and facts and statistics. The clearly written objective narratives provide context and reliable background information. Primary source quotes are carefully selected and cited, exposing the reader to differing points of view. And facts and statistics sections aid the reader in evaluating perspectives. Presenting these key types of information creates a richer, more balanced learning experience.

For better understanding and convenience, the series enhances information by organizing it into narrower topics and adding design features that make it easy for a reader to identify desired content. For example, in *Compact Research: Illegal Immigration*, a chapter covering the economic impact of illegal immigration has an objective narrative explaining the various ways the economy is impacted, a balanced section of numerous primary source quotes on the topic, followed by facts and full-color illustrations to encourage evaluation of contrasting perspectives.

The ancient Roman philosopher Lucius Annaeus Seneca wrote, "It is quality rather than quantity that matters." More than just a collection of content, the *Compact Research* series is simply committed to creating, finding, organizing, and presenting the most relevant and appropriate amount of information on a current topic in a user-friendly style that invites, intrigues, and fosters understanding.

Herpes at a Glance

Herpes Defined

Herpes is a common, highly contagious disease. Each year, millions of adults, adolescents, and children become infected with herpes viruses.

Herpes Virus Types

There are eight types of viruses in the herpes family. Two of these viruses, called herpes simplex type 1 and type 2, cause oral and genital herpes, respectively.

Symptoms

People with herpes can experience mild or severe pain, tingling sensations, itching, fever, or sores around the mouth, face, and genital areas.

An Unpredictable Virus

The herpes virus acts unpredictably in the human body and lasts forever. It may lie dormant for long periods and become active at any time.

Prevalence

Approximately 70 percent of Americans over age 12 have the most common form of herpes, oral herpes. Genital herpes is less common, affecting about 1 in 5 adults and adolescents.

How Herpes Spreads

Herpes simplex virus is usually spread via direct skin-to-skin contact with an infected individual. Oral herpes is most often spread by the exchange of saliva, such as from kissing. Genital herpes is transmitted primarily through sexual intercourse and oral sex.

Preventing the Spread

There are a number of ways to help prevent the spread of herpes: avoiding having sex with or kissing someone who may have herpes; using condoms during sex; avoiding contact with cold sores; and proper hygiene such as washing hands.

Health Effects

Herpes can result in moderate to severe pain and discomfort and in some cases lead to serious illnesses.

Herpes Tests

Many people with herpes will not show any symptoms, and it can be easy to mistake oral herpes or genital herpes for other ailments. Physicians can perform a number of tests to determine accurately whether someone is infected with herpes.

Treatment

Though there is no cure for herpes, several effective prescription drugs have been developed. Also helpful are over-the-counter medications, natural remedies, nutritious diets, proper hygiene, and strengthening the immune system.

Seeking a Vaccine

For years researchers have tried to develop an effective herpes vaccine. To date, no herpes vaccine has been approved for patients.

Overview

❝It is often devastating to receive a diagnosis of herpes.❞

—Stephani Cox, a lead clinician for Planned Parenthood of Illinois.

❝Either by the natural progression of the disease or by therapeutic interventions, herpes is far from a hopeless condition.❞

—Will Whittington, a research investigator with the Sexually Transmitted Diseases Division at the Centers for Disease Control and Prevention.

When Holly Becker was 17, she began dating Derek, a 22-year-old coworker. About a month into the relationship, they had sex for the first time. Derek assured her that he had no sexually transmitted diseases. "He didn't get specific about when he was last tested," says Holly. "I still asked him to wear a condom."[1] Holly noticed that during sex, Derek did not use a condom. Feeling embarrassed and afraid of being rejected, she did not stop him.

Soon Holly experienced pains she had not had before, but she continued to have unprotected sex with Derek. "I wasn't serious with him; we were very casual, so I didn't say anything," she writes. "I figured there was no way I could get anything serious, like herpes, HIV, or syphilis. I was also nervous. I'd never been to a gynecologist, just to my doctor for checkups, and I was too afraid to tell my mother what I was doing."[2] A few months later, her symptoms were unbearable and the pain got worse. Holly could not urinate without screaming out loud. Abdominal pain brought tears to her eyes. One day at work she got very sick. She finally told her mother about the pain and they went to a gynecologist the next morning.

"Thank God for my supportive mother," says Holly. "She held my hand while I screamed in pain as the doctor took a Pap smear and culture. It felt like torture. Imagine this: your entire insides are swollen and inflamed, and someone puts just a slight amount of pressure on that swelling and inflammation. It feels like someone just rammed a sword into you. I have never felt anything so horrible." After seeing the open lesions, her doctor said that there was a good chance that she had genital herpes. Holly concluded, "He must be wrong; he's just trying to scare me. Am I the type of girl who gets herpes?"[3]

What Is Herpes?

Genital herpes, which is what Holly had contracted from her boyfriend, is caused by the herpes simplex virus (HSV), which belongs to the Herpesviridae family of related viruses. Besides herpes simplex, the family consists of six other herpes viruses, including the Epstein-Barr virus, which causes infectious mononucleosis, and varicella zoster, which causes chicken pox in children and shingles in adults.

References to herpes date as far back as ancient Greek times. Hippocrates, the ancient Greek physician known as the father of Western medicine, is known to have written about the appearance of herpes lesions on the skin. In fact, the word *herpes* comes from the Greek word *herpein*, meaning "to creep or crawl," referring to the spreading nature of herpes skin sores.

There are two herpes simplex viruses: oral herpes (type 1) and genital herpes (type 2). Both are common, highly contagious diseases; additionally, genital herpes is a prevalent sexually transmitted disease (STD).

> **After infection, the virus can lie inactive, or dormant, for short or very long periods of time, and then become reactivated at any time.**

Of the two simplex viruses, oral herpes (also called HSV-1) is more common in humans than genital herpes (HSV-2). Under a microscope both viruses are virtually identical, sharing approximately 50 percent of their genetic makeup.

Herpes simplex causes blisters and sores, or ulcers, on the skin. The

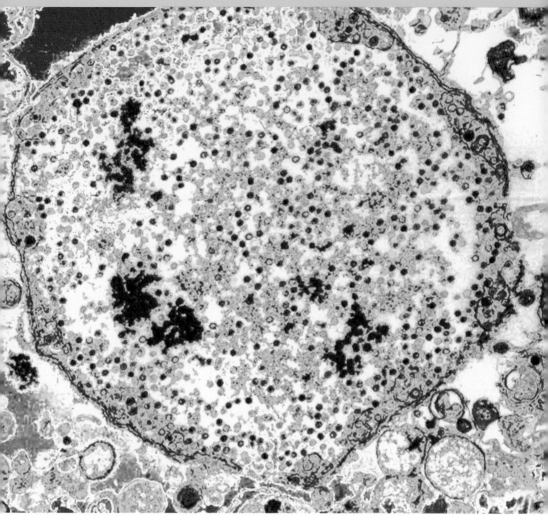

Herpes simplex type 1, the virus that causes cold sores, can be seen in this colored transmission electron micrograph of a section of a cell. Tiny spherical virus particles (dark blue) fill the cell and can be seen emerging from it (lower right) to infect other cells.

virus enters the body through breaks in the skin or through the skin of the mouth or genitals. Once within the body, herpes infects the ganglia, which are groups of nerve cell bodies. After infection, the virus can lie inactive, or dormant, for short or very long periods of time, and then become reactivated at any time.

Herpes is a DNA-type virus, inserting its DNA—or genetic makeup—directly into the nerve endings of the skin, which then leads along nerve fibers to the nucleus of the nerve cell. The viruses then begin making copies of their viral particles and spread elsewhere, which can lead to recurring herpes outbreaks. Thus, the herpes virus remains in the body forever, going through stages of dormancy and activity. No cure for herpes currently exists.

Symptoms of Herpes Infection

Sores caused by herpes simplex can develop on almost any area of the skin but usually appear around the face and genitals. Symptoms can include itching, rash, sores, blisters, painful burning, and swollen glands. The first outbreak, known as the primary outbreak, is often accompanied by fever and headaches, fatigue, and swollen lymph nodes. Herpes viruses act unpredictably in individuals, so outbreaks and symptoms may be mild, severe, recurring, or perhaps never appear. According to the American Social Health Association, "A person may show symptoms within days after contracting genital herpes, or it may take weeks, months, or years."[4]

Men and women with type 1 oral herpes can get cold sores—also known as fever blisters—on the lips, gums, tongue, nose, inside or outside of the mouth, and around the face and eyes. People with type 2 genital herpes may experience inflamed blisters and sores around their genital areas.

In men genital herpes sores usually appear on or around the penis and scrotum. In women the sores can be present in the vagina, on the cervix, or on the labia. Both sexes may also be affected in or around the anus. Infection of

> **It is quite common for people with genital herpes to show no symptoms or to have symptoms so mild they may not recognize them.**

the male or female urethra frequently causes a burning sensation when urinating. Other symptoms may include muscle aches, swollen glands in the groin area, and discharge from the vagina or penis.

These symptoms are not always easy to identify as herpes related because other conditions are sometimes confused with herpes. For example, canker sores, which are caused by a variety of factors but are not

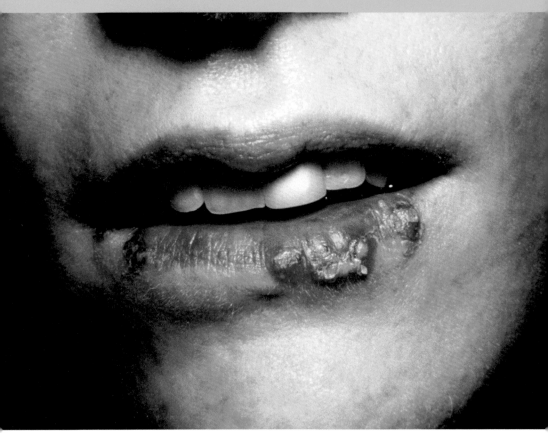

Oral herpes, one of two forms of the herpes simplex virus, results most often in painful sores on the lips, gums, or tongue. The other form of the virus is genital herpes. Both are common, uncomfortable, and highly contagious.

contagious, may be mistaken for oral herpes. Similarly, yeast infections, which are commonplace irritations of the vagina caused by excess yeast, may be mistaken for genital herpes. It is quite common for people with genital herpes to show no symptoms or to have symptoms so mild they may not recognize them. As pathologist and medical journalist Melissa Conrad Stöppler writes, "As many as 80%–90% of those infected fail to recognize genital herpes symptoms or have no symptoms at all."[5]

Testing for Herpes

A doctor usually can diagnose genital herpes based on a physical exam and the results of certain laboratory tests. To aid in detection of herpes, a doctor or health professional will often ask patients about their sexual history. A doctor may then have lab tests performed on blood, lesion cells, or fluids. There are several different herpes tests, with varying degrees of accuracy.

Tests are available for both types of herpes simplex, but most testing is done for genital herpes. A common procedure is a culture test, in which a physician takes a tissue sample by scraping cells from an open sore. Doctors can also use blood tests to detect the presence of herpes simplex virus antibodies, which develop in a person's blood to fight the infection. According to the American Social Health Association, blood tests are recommended after 12 to 16 weeks from the time of possible exposure.

Who Is Affected?

Each year, millions of adults, adolescents, and even young children are newly infected with one of the herpes simplex viruses. About 70 percent of Americans over age 12—approximately 100 million people—have oral herpes, the more common form of herpes simplex. Most people contract oral herpes as children when receiving a kiss from an infected relative or friend, not through sexual contact. Oral herpes can be spread quite easily among people through skin-to-skin contact.

Genital herpes—affecting about 1 in 6 adolescents and adults—is one of the most common STDs in America, according to the Centers for Disease Control and Prevention (CDC). Though it is less common than oral herpes, genital herpes infects approximately half a million to 1 million Americans each year. An estimated 45 million to 50 million Americans ages 12 and older have genital herpes.

In rare cases newborns can acquire genital herpes from their mothers, which is called neonatal herpes. Approximately, 1,000 to 3,000 newborns are thus affected each year in the United States out of a total of 4 million births. Infants may suffer serious neurological damage, mental retardation, or death as a result of neonatal herpes infections. In the vast major-

> " Though it is less common than oral herpes, genital herpes infects approximately half a million to 1 million Americans each year. "

ity of such cases, neonatal herpes is transmitted when an infant comes into contact with the herpes virus in the birth canal during delivery. If a mother does have lesions or herpes symptoms during pregnancy, the safest practice is a cesarean delivery. This prevents the baby from coming into contact with active virus.

What Are the Health Effects of Herpes?

Herpes simplex is rarely life threatening, but it can lead to potentially serious physical conditions and illness. In some cases of oral herpes, infection can occur in the eye, causing what is known as ocular herpes. Approximately 50,000 Americans develop this condition each year. This infection can cause eye redness, tearing, swelling, and more serious problems such as blurred vision and scarring of the cornea (a leading cause of blindness). In very rare cases oral herpes can spread to the brain, causing herpes encephalitis, a dangerous infection that can result in death or long-term brain damage. Oral herpes has also been identified as the cause of most cases of Bell's palsy, a facial nerve paralysis that affects approximately 40,000 Americans each year.

Herpes outbreaks can often be uncomfortable and painful. In the words of Heather Brannon, a family practice physician, "The first genital herpes outbreak is more painful and lasts longer than recurrent genital herpes outbreaks in both men and women."[6] Many experts point out that because of the female anatomy, women are at a much higher risk of being infected than men. This is because a woman's genital area has a greater number of mucosal cells—cells containing body fluids—which are a main entry point for the herpes virus.

One worrisome aspect of genital herpes, according to researchers, is the role it may play in the spread of HIV, the virus that causes AIDS. According to the CDC, "Herpes can make people more susceptible to HIV infection, and it can make HIV-infected individuals more infectious."[7] The CDC points to studies showing that heterosexuals with genital herpes are twice as much at risk for HIV as those who are not infected.

How Herpes Spreads

Herpes simplex viruses spread from person to person through skin-to-skin contact, most often through kissing or sexual contact with an infected person. Herpes is most infectious during the period when itchy sores start to appear on the skin during an outbreak. But even if an outbreak causes no visible symptoms or breaks in the skin, there is still a risk of the virus being passed on to another person through skin contact. When an infected person is asymptomatic—or not showing symptoms—oral or genital herpes could still be transmitted to another person.

Oral herpes is spread primarily from the exchange of saliva by kissing. Even just a friendly kiss on the cheek can spread the herpes virus if one of the people involved has an open herpes sore. In many cases a parent will transmit—often unknowingly—oral herpes to a child via kissing.

Genital herpes is spread via sexual contact. According to the American Congress of Obstetricians and Gynecologists: "The herpes virus can pass through a break in your skin during vaginal, oral, or anal sex. It can enter the moist membranes of the penis, vagina, urinary opening, cervix, or anus."[8] The herpes virus enters the body through the thin skin of the genital area and travels along a nerve pathway to a bundle of nerves at the base of the

> " In very rare cases oral herpes can spread to the brain, causing herpes encephalitis, a dangerous infection that can result in death or long-term brain damage. "

spine called the dorsal root ganglion. There it remains inactive, causing no harm and no symptoms, until something triggers it to "wake up" and become active. Sometimes, the triggers may be stress, lack of sleep, fever, sun exposure, or menstruation. At other times, there may appear to be no reason at all for the virus to become active.

Herpes cannot be transmitted from toilet seats, shared straws, toothbrushes, bath towels, or utensils. Because the herpes virus requires a living host cell to survive, it cannot exist for very long outside the body.

How Can Herpes Be Treated?

Many drugs, treatments, and remedies are available to treat people infected with herpes. Foremost are three antiviral prescription drugs that are approved by the U.S. Food and Drug Administration for the treatment of oral and genital herpes: acyclovir, famciclovir, and valacyclovir.

Usually taken orally, these drugs have been found to be effective in reducing the symptoms and frequency of sores and blisters in patients. These three drugs may also be useful in treating those people who are prone to frequent outbreaks of herpes.

> " **Oral herpes is spread primarily from the exchange of saliva by kissing. Even just a friendly kiss on the cheek can spread the herpes virus if one of the people involved has an open herpes sore.** "

Two types of treatment using these antiviral drugs can be helpful to people with herpes. The first is episodic treatment, beginning at the first warning signs of an outbreak, such as itching or tingling, and continuing for several days. Episodic therapy helps to shorten the duration of symptoms and to speed the healing of sores, but it may do little to reduce the frequency of attacks. Reducing outbreaks is the goal of the second treatment, suppressive therapy. With this therapy, patients who are susceptible to frequently recurring outbreaks take antiviral drugs daily for long periods of time, usually lasting from several months to a year. Suppressive therapy is also helpful in preventing the transmission of herpes from an infected person to an uninfected sexual partner.

Once oral or genital herpes symptoms appear, other medicines such as aspirin, ibuprofen, and acetaminophen can be beneficial. These can reduce fever, headaches, pain from sores, and swelling in the genital area.

Coping with Herpes

Many people are shocked when they show signs of herpes or are diagnosed by a doctor. Because symptoms often take a long time to develop, many infected people may be puzzled as to when or from whom they contracted the virus. Individuals also may feel embarrassed about visible signs of their outbreaks or telling their partners that they have herpes. Some people with genital herpes may view their infection as a taboo subject; they may be uncomfortable discussing the disease with people close to them.

Single men and women with herpes may feel limited from dating or pursuing serious relationships. They may fear infecting another person or feel afraid of rejection if they admit that they have herpes. In the words of psychologist Jerry Kennard, "For people with genital herpes, the shame and fear of isolation that can accompany the virus may even affect their decision to tell sexual partners."[9]

In long-term relationships or marriages, issues of mistrust often arise when one partner is diagnosed with herpes. One person may believe that the infected partner had sex outside the relationship. But since signs of genital herpes may take a very long time to appear, it is often impossible to tell which partner actually contracted the disease first.

The advice from many people who have written about herpes and relationships is for people to be open and up front about the disease. They stress that telling new partners about one's herpes infection is the best approach to take for the sake of both partners.

How Can the Spread of Herpes Be Prevented?

Herpes is a very contagious disease. However, acting cautiously can help reduce the spread of herpes. For example, people who experience an outbreak should not touch visible sores or break open blisters. They should also be careful of, or avoid, facial or body contact with others, including kissing and sex. It is important to wash hands thoroughly with soap if a sore is touched.

Herpes is most contagious when sores or blisters are present. But even when sores are not visible, the viruses can still be transmitted to other people. Also, medical professionals caution that if one person has oral herpes, he or she could potentially transmit the virus during oral sex and cause genital herpes in the other partner.

> " Because symptoms often take a long time to develop, many infected people may be puzzled as to when or from whom they contracted the virus. "

Therefore, experts advocate taking certain measures to avoid the spread of herpes, such as abstaining from sex, practicing monogamous sex with an uninfected partner, and avoiding any sex during herpes outbreaks. The spread of herpes can be further reduced by using condoms or dental dams, which protect against the virus during oral sex. Many experts agree that prevention efforts can be more effective if more people learn the facts about herpes and take correct precautionary steps.

Thwarting the Herpes Virus

For years virologists have been studying ways to protect uninfected people from the herpes virus. In 2002 the National Institute of Allergy and Infectious Diseases and the drug company GlaxoSmithKline began clinical trials for a vaccine called Herpevac (now called Simplirix). The vaccine was tested on more than 7,000 women who had neither oral herpes nor genital herpes. Results showed the vaccine to be only partially effective, and further research was planned.

While the United States is one of several countries studying herpes vaccines, no vaccine has yet been approved for use in this country. Similarly, researchers in the United States and abroad are aiming to produce creams or foams with microbicides that could kill or disable herpes viruses. Women and men could then apply such products to their genital areas before sex, thus protecting themselves from herpes infection.

Increasingly, scientists are making more discoveries about how the herpes virus acts within the body's cells, nerve paths, and tissues and what might be required to combat it. As scientific understanding about herpes viruses progresses, many people look forward to a day when modern medicine renders the disease harmless in the body or finds a cure to vanquish herpes altogether.

What Is Herpes?

> **Herpes simplex virus (HSV) affects more than one third of the world's population and is responsible for a wide array of human disease, with effects ranging from discomfort to death.**
>
> —David H. Emmert, a family physician in Millersville, Pennsylvania.

> **If you have HSV, you have in your body a virus that operates, in most ways, just like dozens of other viruses you've carried around from time to time. The trouble with herpes simplex is that your immune system can't completely get rid of it.**
>
> —Charles Ebel and Anna Wald, authors of *Managing Herpes: Living and Loving with HSV.*

For centuries humankind has been aware of skin infections related to herpes, even if the cause was not known. Descriptions of herpes lesions were found on a Sumerian tablet from 3000 B.C. The Ebers Papyrus, an Egyptian medical document from around 1500 B.C., prescribed treatment for oral herpes. In A.D. 1736 genital herpes was first described by Jean Astruc, a physician to King Louis XIV of France, although he did not assign a name to the condition.

In the early 1800s English physicians Robert Willan and Thomas Bateman made the first clear distinction between "herpes labialis" (oral herpes) and "herpes praeputialis" (genital herpes). It was not until 1893, however, that French dermatologist Jean Baptiste Emile Vidal made the breakthrough discovery that herpes was indeed infectious.

Thereafter, doctors and scientists gradually learned more and more about the causes and effects of herpes. Still, it was difficult to pinpoint exactly what it was that caused painful sores and lesions to break out on people's faces and bodies—or why. More importantly, as journalist John Leo explained in a 1982 *Time* magazine cover story, "So little known was the virus that doctors confidently misdiagnosed it right up through the late 1970s."[10] Indeed, it was not until the end of the 1960s that scientists confirmed the existence of two separate herpes simplex viruses: oral herpes and genital herpes.

> " Two of the herpes viruses, known as herpes simplex, are extremely contagious and can cause infectious sores around the face and genitals—and potentially anywhere on a person's skin. "

Herpes is actually a large group of viruses that belong to the Herpesviridae family of viruses, which causes diseases in people and animals. Eight of these viruses affect humans, causing diseases such as chicken pox, shingles, mononucleosis, and others. Herpes viruses are a leading cause of human viral disease, behind only the common cold and influenza viruses. Two of the herpes viruses, known as herpes simplex, are extremely contagious and can cause infectious sores around the face and genitals—and potentially anywhere on a person's skin.

How the Herpes Virus Acts

Like all other viruses, herpes simplex depends on a living host cell in order to reproduce. The virus cannot penetrate normal, healthy layers of skin, so it enters the body through cracks or breaks in the skin. It also enters through mucous membranes such as the mouth, vagina, rectum, tip of the penis, or the eye. At these sites, the virus will attack surface skin cells.

Herpes viruses are very small compared to the cells they infect. They use a protein on their exterior to locate and bind to a host cell. They then inject their genetic material into the host cell, taking control and using that cell's DNA to reproduce and churn out viruses by the millions. The cells become so full that they eventually rupture and die, releasing more viruses to infect surrounding cells. This destruction of the host cells is responsible for the characteristic signs and symptoms of herpes outbreaks, such as sores, clusters of blisters, or rashes.

When the herpes virus is not busy reproducing, it "hides" in nerve root cells, where it lies inactive in what is called a latent state. In the case of oral herpes, the virus hides in the trigeminal ganglion, a bundle of nerve tissue in the brain that allows for feeling and movement of the mouth and parts of the face. With genital herpes, the virus retreats to the sacral ganglion, located at the base of the spine. This evasive tactic allows the virus to escape detection by the body's immune system, waiting for an ideal opportunity to cause a new outbreak. As authors Charles Ebel and Anna Wald write, "The defining event of infection is latency—the virus's successful effort to set up a permanent base of operations."[11]

Two Types of Herpes

There are two types of herpes simplex virus, HSV-1 and HSV-2 (also called type 1 and type 2), and it can be easy to confuse them with each other. In fact, both viruses are nearly identical, sharing approximately 50 percent of their genetic makeup. The primary difference between them is their "site of preference," or where the viruses are likely to cause infection. The HSV-1 virus is responsible for nearly all oral herpes infections (oral herpes from HSV-2 is rare). The vast majority of genital herpes infections are caused by the HSV-2 virus.

It is important to realize, however, that a person infected with HSV-1 is capable of transmitting genital herpes to a partner by performing oral sex. Terri Warren, an STD clinician and author, notes that HSV-1 now accounts for almost 40 percent of new genital herpes infections in America. As Warren points out, "In teens and college students, HSV-1 accounts for even more new herpes cases than HSV-2, probably because of the popularity of oral sex among young

> " It is important to realize, however, that a person infected with HSV-1 is capable of transmitting genital herpes to a partner by performing oral sex. "

people."[12] While HSV-1 is the more common of the two viruses among people of all ages, HSV-2 is responsible for the majority of recurring herpes outbreaks.

Unpredictable by Nature

Herpes is a disease well known for its unpredictability. It can range from an unnoticeable "silent" virus to a chronic ordeal involving excruciating pain. Latency can last for months, perhaps even years. People with herpes, and doctors themselves, cannot forecast when outbreaks will occur, what factors might trigger them, or even how severe they may be. Symptoms vary with each individual, from mild to very painful, and they may not appear for weeks or months after infection occurs. While many people are fortunate to have only one or two outbreaks in a lifetime, others may experience more than the average of five recurrences a year. It can be quite puzzling that the same virus that causes no symptoms for one person (asymptomatic infection) may cause very painful symptoms in his or her partner.

When someone has a herpes outbreak, it is nearly impossible to pinpoint exactly what prompts the virus to activate. Experts point to a weakened immune system as one factor that plays a major role. As Gayla Baer McCord, a creator of herpes support groups, writes, "Having a weakened immune system does not cause the virus to become stronger, it simply makes the body less able to cope with the virus that is there."[13] When it does reactivate, the virus will usually target that part of the body where the infection first occurred. Migrating from the nerve tissues, the herpes virus travels along nerve pathways and sets a course for the surface skin cells. In doing so, it produces warning signs—itching, tingling, numbness, or burning—that the virus is becoming active.

> " The first symptoms of cold sores may include pain around the mouth and on the lips, fever, a sore throat, muscle aches, or swollen glands in the neck or other parts of the body. "

Once the virus reaches the skin, a cluster of small blisters (also called sores or lesions) may form, filled with clear or whitish fluid. Eventually, the blisters rupture, turning into ulcers—open sores that ooze fluid or bleed. Medical professionals warn that this is the most contagious phase of an outbreak. Over a 7- to 14-day period, the ulcers will dry up and turn into crusty scabs, indicating the end of an outbreak. The scabs eventually break off, and the healing process usually leaves the skin unscarred. The period from first symptoms to the final healing stage lasts about 1 to 2 weeks for oral herpes and 2 to 4 weeks for genital herpes.

> **As with oral herpes, initial outbreaks of genital herpes are usually more painful and last longer than recurring outbreaks.**

Oral Herpes

Most oral herpes infections occur before adulthood. Children will frequently contract the disease when kissed by parents, relatives, or friends. Usually, infected saliva comes into contact with soft tissue around the mouth, or the contagious area touches cracks or breaks in the skin of a child's face.

Oral herpes can cause sores almost anywhere around the face, but usually around the mouth or on the lips. Facial blisters are often referred to as cold sores or fever blisters, and their number can vary from one to several. The first symptoms of cold sores may include pain around the mouth and on the lips, fever, a sore throat, muscle aches, or swollen glands in the neck or other parts of the body. The skin around the blisters is often red, swollen, and sore. Besides the mouth and lips, sores can form on the gums, the front of the tongue, the inside of the cheeks, the throat, and the roof of the mouth.

Initial oral herpes outbreaks (primary infections) are often more painful and longer lasting than recurring outbreaks, because the body has not yet produced neutralizing antibodies and other natural defenses to combat the virus. Primary infections can be especially troublesome for young children, who may get oral herpes even as infants. Pediatric dentist Daniel Ravel explains:

The symptoms of this initial infection are painful for infants and toddlers. Blisters form on the tongue and palate. The child's gums (gingiva) appear fiery red and are painful to the touch. Infected children easily become dehydrated and weak, due to the pain associated with eating and drinking. Toddlers with primary herpes experience fever, malaise, loss of appetite, and severe intraoral pain.[14]

It is estimated that approximately one-half to two-thirds of American teens and adults have oral herpes, although the vast majority will not develop sores.

Genital Herpes

Genital herpes is one of the most common sexually transmitted diseases reported each year. The disease is spread by intercourse, oral sex, anal sex, or skin-to-skin contact. Outbreaks are often preceded by warning signs such as headache, fever, lower back pain, burning sensation in the genitals, pain when urinating, and tender lumps in the groin area. Among men, sores typically develop on the glans (end of the penis), the foreskin, and shaft of the penis, as well as on the scrotum. Women will develop sores on the vulva, vagina, or cervix. People with genital herpes may also get sores near their genitals. As authors Ebel and Wald explain:

> A man might experience lesions on the penis the first several times he has an outbreak, for example, and then discover herpes lesions on his buttock or upper thigh the next time. Overall, about 20% of people will have a nongenital herpes recurrence, and the buttocks and legs are the most likely sites for such recurrences.[15]

Both men and women may also find it painful to urinate if lesions develop near the urethra.

The number of outbreaks and the degree of pain associated with genital herpes varies from person to person. Many factors come into play, such as site of the infection, whether it is an initial or recurring outbreak, and the overall health of the individual. As with oral herpes, initial outbreaks of genital herpes are usually more painful and last longer than recurring outbreaks. Consider the case of Edward, a 33-year-old gym owner, who contracted genital herpes prior to getting married. Edward reports that he has about 8 to 12 outbreaks per year, usually with aching in the groin and legs. He says that after he infected his wife, she had a terrible initial outbreak but experienced no other outbreaks for 7 years.

Experts contend that even though people may go long periods without outbreaks, it is quite common for the herpes virus to appear on the skin without symptoms. This phenomenon—known as asymptomatic shedding—is considered to be responsible for the majority of genital herpes cases. According to the California Department of Public Health, "All people infected with HSV-2 shed the virus asymptomatically, regardless of a history of symptomatic recurrences, thus the sexual contacts of individuals with symptomatic or asymptomatic HSV-2 are at risk of becoming infected."[16] One perplexing aspect is that asymptomatic shedding can occur at any time without anyone knowing where on the infected person's body it is taking place.

How Many Affected

According to the CDC, nearly 20 million Americans are infected with genital herpes, with approximately a half-million new cases reported each year. Experts estimate that a similar number of new cases goes unreported. The CDC's National Health and Nutrition Examination Survey released in March 2010 found that 16 percent of the population between the ages of 14 and 49 had genital herpes. The survey also confirmed what many researchers had theorized for many years: Nearly 80 percent of people who have genital herpes have not been diagnosed and may not know they have the disease.

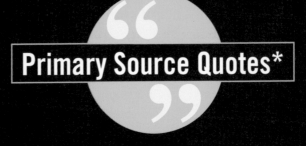

Primary Source Quotes*

What Is Herpes?

66 Herpes is looked on with horror by many people with new infection or who are worried about getting herpes. 99

—H. Hunter Handsfield, "Genital Herpes: Framing the Problem, Diagnosing the Disease," October 4, 2007. http://cme.medscape.com

Handsfield is a clinical professor of medicine at the University of Washington in Seattle.

66 When herpes 'wakes' and travels to the surface of the skin or mucous membranes, it is often subtle and hard to recognize, even for a health care provider, and sometimes impossible to spot. 99

—American Social Health Association, "Learn About Herpes," 2010. www.ashastd.org.

The American Social Health Association is a nonprofit public health organization in North Carolina.

* Editor's Note: While the definition of a primary source can be narrowly or broadly defined, for the purposes of Compact Research, a primary source consists of: 1) results of original research presented by an organization or researcher; 2) eyewitness accounts of events, personal experience, or work experience; 3) first-person editorials offering pundits' opinions; 4) government officials presenting political plans and/or policies; 5) representatives of organizations presenting testimony or policy.

❝Most people (85%) with genital herpes will have recurring outbreaks—sometimes 6 to 10 a year.❞

—Melissa Conrad Stöppler, "Genital Herpes," eMedicineHealth, August 19, 2009. www.emedicinehealth.com.

Stöppler is a specialist consultant in the breast oncology research program at the University of California–San Francisco School of Medicine.

❝In 70 percent of patients, transmission or spreading the disease happened when the person known to have HSV had no symptoms!❞

—Lois McGuire, "Herpes Symptoms, Diagnosis and How It Spreads," MayoClinic.com, December 5, 2008. www.mayoclinic.com.

McGuire is a nurse practitioner at the Mayo Clinic in Rochester, Minnesota.

❝Historically, it was thought that herpes could only be spread if you had sex with a person with an outbreak—with open lesions. However, that theory was blown out of the water several years ago with the discovery of a phenomenon called viral shedding.❞

—Charlotte Grayson, "Transmitting Herpes: How to Protect the Ones You Love," Health Central, 2010. www.healthcentral.com.

Grayson practices internal medicine in Fayetteville, Georgia.

❝The only [thing] that's been scientifically proven to be a trigger is extended periods of stress lasting more than two weeks.❞

—Terri Warren, *The Good News About the Bad News: Herpes; Everything You Need to Know*. Oakland, CA: New Harbinger, 2009.

Warren operates the Westover Heights Clinic, a private clinic in Portland, Oregon, specializing in the diagnosis and treatment of sexually transmitted diseases.

❝I don't think even many doctors know how common genital herpes is.❞

—Edward Hook, "Herpes Awareness Project Divides Health Officials," *Washington Post*, July 24, 2007.

Hook is an infectious disease specialist at the University of Alabama–Birmingham.

....

❝It is estimated that 20 percent of people with genital herpes will never have symptoms in their lifetimes and that 80 percent will—although most of them will not realize that their symptoms are from herpes.❞

—Lisa Marr, *Sexually Transmitted Diseases: A Physician Tells You What You Need to Know*. Baltimore, MD: Johns Hopkins University Press, 2007.

Marr practices geriatric medicine in Milwaukee, Wisconsin.

....

❝Twenty to thirty percent of U.S. adults are believed to have HSV-2 antibodies. That percent is pretty high. Without doubt, most of those people are unaware of being infected.❞

—Go Ask Alice, "Testing for Asymptomatic Herpes," June 30, 2008 www.goaskalice.columbia.edu.

Go Ask Alice is a Columbia University program that helps its students access health information and resources.

....

Facts and Illustrations

What Is Herpes?

- It is estimated that from **500,000 to 1 million** Americans are infected with genital herpes each year.

- According to the Centers for Disease Control and Prevention, **16.2 percent** of Americans 14 to 49 years of age—about 1 in 6—has genital herpes.

- **Touching** any type of herpes sore may spread the virus from one partner to another.

- The oral herpes virus can also cause genital herpes; it is often transmitted by **oral-to-genital contact**.

- If someone has **oral and genital sex** with an infected partner, he or she can acquire the infection at both sites.

- According to a Centers for Disease Control and Prevention survey, a decrease in newly diagnosed genital herpes cases from **21 percent to 17 percent** was found during the years 1999 to 2004.

- Nearly **twice as many women** as men are found to be infected with genital herpes.

- According to the Mayo Clinic, up to **90 percent** of people infected with herpes are unaware that they have the disease.

Genital Herpes by Sex and Age Group

Genital herpes is more common among U.S. women than men and prevalence increases with age, according to the U.S. Centers for Disease Control and Prevention. Studies show that overall, 20.9 percent of women and 11.5 percent of men have HSV-2 in the United States. The prevalence of genital herpes is highest among men and women aged 40-49. The CDC monitors total cases of genital herpes and rates of new infection through the National Health and Nutrition Examination Survey (NHANES).

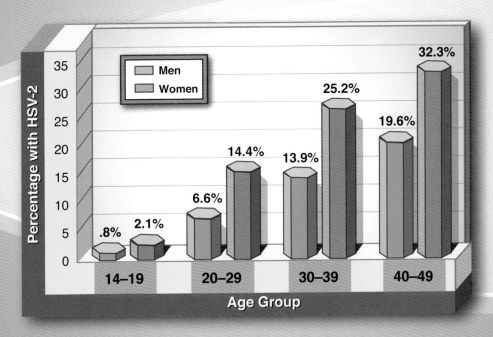

Source: Centers for Disease Control and Prevention, "National Health and Nutrition Examination Survey, United States, 2005–2008," *Morbidity and Mortality Weekly Report*, April 23, 2010. www.cdc.gov.

- If a person tests positive for genital herpes but has **never had symptoms**, it cannot be determined how long the virus has been present, when or whether they will have outbreaks, or whether the virus will ever cause a problem.

Genital Herpes by Age and Race/Ethnicity

Genital herpes is approximately 3 times more common among U.S. blacks than whites and nearly 4 times that of Mexican Americans, with the highest prevalence among blacks between the ages of 30 and 49, according to the U.S. Centers for Disease Control and Prevention. Study results show that overall, 39.2 percent of African Americans are infected with genital herpes compared with 12.3 percent of whites and 10.1 percent of Mexican Americans. The CDC monitors total cases of genital herpes and rates of new infection through the National Health and Nutrition Examination Survey (NHANES).

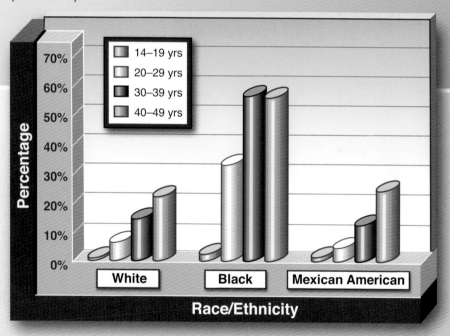

Source: Centers for Disease Control and Prevention, "National Health and Nutrition Examination Survey, United States, 2005–2008," *Morbidity and Mortality Weekly Report*, April 23, 2010. www.cdc.gov.

- It is estimated that **1 to 3 percent** of individuals with asymptomatic genital herpes are shedding the virus at any particular time.

Number of First-Time Cases of Herpes

Genital herpes is not required to be reported to federal health authorities. Each year, private physicians in the United States voluntarily report to the National Disease and Therapeutic Index the number of first-time herpes cases they encounter. Over time, first-time visits to physicians for herpes have increased although the most recent numbers, between 2006 and 2008, show a decrease.

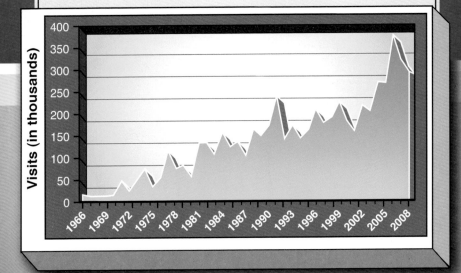

Genital Herpes—Initial visits to physicians' offices: United States, 1966–2008

Source: Centers for Disease Control and Prevention, "Sexually Transmitted Diseases Surveillance, 2008," 2009. www.cdc.gov.

What Are the Health Effects of Herpes?

> **Several dozen complications are already known to be associated with herpes infections of different types, and more are being discovered each year.**
>
> —Dennis Clark, who holds a Ph.D. in plant science from the University of Texas–Austin and specializes in the medicinal qualities of plants.

> **Genital herpes infections do not cause permanent disability or long-term damage in healthy adults. However, in people who have suppressed immune systems, HSV episodes can be long-lasting and unusually severe.**
>
> —Illinois Department of Public Health, which is responsible for protecting the state's residents through the prevention and control of disease and injury.

Although rashes and blisters are commonly associated with herpes infections, there are lesser-known and more serious—even deadly—complications caused by herpes simplex viruses. In November 2007 Charlotte Raveney and Mohamed Eisawy, a married couple in Great Britain, welcomed the birth of their first child, an 8-pound (3.6kg) girl named Mira. After a long and painful labor, Raveney was exhausted. Mira had a slightly sticky eye, but was breast-feeding and seemed to be thriving. Recovering in the hospital three days later, Raveney noticed a cold sore developing on her own bottom lip, the first such sore she had ever had. A hospital midwife assured her it was nothing to worry about and blamed it on the stress of birth and lack of sleep. "She said it would soon disappear, and she was right—the next day it had gone,"[17] Raveney says.

Four days after returning home, Raveney's baby resisted breast-feeding, which lasted only two or three minutes at a time, and was unusually sleepy. A general practitioner examined Mira and prescribed eyedrops for her. The baby was examined again the following day and was pronounced well. But that night, when Eisawy picked Mira up, her body went rigid and she started shaking. Raveney noticed red spots on Mira's stomach. The couple took their baby to the hospital. Soon after arrival Mira stopped breathing and was put on a ventilator.

> " Infants contract herpes viruses in three different ways: while in the uterus (most rare), passing through the birth canal (most common), and soon after birth. "

Four hours later the couple received the heartbreaking news that doctors were unable to help her. Raveney and Eisawy decided to have the ventilator switched off, and 10-day-old Mira died. Five weeks later the couple learned that Mira had died from an oral herpes virus. As Raveney explains: "Apparently, babies are most at risk from this virus during the first six weeks of their life because of their poor immunity. If doctors had known that this was my first ever cold sore, Mira could have been given anti-viral drugs to ensure that the damage was caught and the virus didn't spread."[18]

How Babies Contract Herpes

Most pregnant women with herpes are able to deliver healthy children who are not infected by the virus. In rare cases, however, newborns contract what is known as neonatal herpes, which strikes an estimated 1,000 infants in the United States each year. Left untreated, neonatal herpes can be devastating to infants, causing serious long-term damage or death. Infants contract herpes viruses in three different ways: while in the uterus (most rare), passing through the birth canal (most common), and soon after birth. Neonatal herpes is more likely when women are first infected with herpes during pregnancy, with the risk to the fetus increasing during the final three months. This is because there is a large amount of virus present and insufficient time for a mother to produce antibodies to protect the fetus.

During vaginal birth, babies can contract herpes by coming into contact with active sores in the birth canal. According to authors Charles Ebel and Anna Wald, "It turns out that more than half of the babies infected with herpes at delivery are born to mothers who acquired genital herpes in the last few weeks of pregnancy. Some of these women actually had herpes lesions but did not realize it and were not adequately examined before giving birth."[19] If a mother has such sores prior to delivery, doctors often perform a cesarean delivery or prescribe antiviral drugs to reduce the chance of the baby's infection.

Deadly and Debilitating

The most severe type of neonatal herpes is known as disseminated infection, in which the herpes virus circulates throughout the baby's bloodstream, causing death or severe internal damage. The associated death rate is very high: 85 percent of untreated cases and more than 50 percent of babies who receive treatment. Infants who do survive often experience long-term problems affecting organs such as the brain, heart, kidneys, liver, and lungs.

Another type of deadly birth-acquired herpes is CNS infection which affects the central nervous system, usually causing inflammation of the brain, or encephalitis. Approximately 50 to 70 percent of untreated babies die, while most survivors suffer from long-term neurological complications such as learning disabilities, impaired movement, and blindness as well as low birth weight. Lastly, babies can suffer from localized herpes infections of the skin, eyes, or mouth, creating the small fluid-filled blisters that commonly affect adults. While not immediately life threatening, localized infections are likely to progress to either disseminated or CNS infections without prompt treatment.

> " While not immediately life threatening, localized infections are likely to progress to either disseminated or CNS infections without prompt treatment. "

The Herpes and HIV Link

In 1988 the CDC began to examine the biological interaction between herpes viruses and HIV, the virus that causes AIDS. Since that time several studies have concluded that having HSV-2 genital herpes at least doubles the risk of acquiring HIV. It became evident to scientists why these individuals are at high risk. First, genital herpes—or any infection that causes open sores or breaks in the skin—creates a portal for HIV to enter the body. Therefore, someone with genital herpes sores can become infected if their sores come into contact with the blood, semen, or vaginal secretions of an HIV-infected person. Second, the white blood cells (T lymphocytes) that the body calls on to combat herpes viruses are the very same cells that are targeted by the HIV virus.

Just as herpes viruses seek host cells to replicate, HIV invades T lymphocyte cells by attaching to proteins called CD4 located on the cell surface. According to Lawrence Corey, the lead investigator of a 2009 study funded by the National Institute of Allergy and Infectious Diseases, even long after genital herpes sores had healed, extremely high concentrations of T lymphocytes surrounded the affected tissue, providing ample opportunities for HIV infection. As Corey writes: "We hypothesized that sores and breaks in the skin from HSV-2 are associated with a long-lasting immune response at those locations, and that the response consists of an influx of cells that are a perfect storm for HIV infection. We believe HIV gains access to these cells mainly through microscopic breaks in the skin that occur during sex."[20]

> "Persons infected with both genital herpes and HIV may get more frequent herpes outbreaks, longer-lasting outbreaks, and more severe outbreaks with larger blisters."

Infected with Both Diseases

Researchers have long known that most HIV-infected individuals—perhaps 60 to 70 percent—are also infected with HSV-2 genital herpes. People who are coinfected carry severe health burdens compared to others who are infected with HIV alone. For example, persons infected with both genital herpes and HIV may get more frequent herpes outbreaks, longer-lasting outbreaks, and more severe outbreaks with larger blisters. In 2004 researchers Corey, Wald, and others wrote, "In the setting of untreated, advanced HIV-1 disease, HSV ulcers are often large, deep . . . slow to heal, often appear in atypical areas of the body, and can lead to scarring."[21] Treating people infected with both herpes and HIV could provide a boost that their immune systems need so that genital herpes outbreaks occur less frequently and are less severe.

Coinfected individuals are also at risk of their HIV developing into AIDS at a more rapid rate. Studies have shown that frequent genital herpes recurrences increase the amount of HIV in the blood and genital tract and are a factor in the development of AIDS. In 2001 Timothy Schacker, a Minneapolis physician and researcher at the University of Minnesota, wrote that "a significant predictor of rapid onset of AIDS in persons with a high CD4-positive cell count was reactivation of HSV in the year prior to the onset of AIDS. The reason for this may be that HSV-2 reactivation somehow drives the rate of HIV-1 replication higher."[22]

Some Promising News

In 2010 a study published in the *New England Journal of Medicine* announced promising news to individuals infected with both genital herpes and HIV. Over the course of 2 years, researchers at 14 sites across Africa studied 3,400 heterosexual couples in which 1 partner was infected with both herpes and HIV and the other was not. Half the participants were treated with an antiviral drug called acyclovir, and the other half received a placebo.

The researchers found that genital herpes outbreaks were 73 percent lower among the acyclovir group compared with the placebo group. This study also found that the amount of HIV present in the blood and genital tracts of the acyclovir group decreased twofold. The result confirmed the outcome of five earlier studies that had shown it is possible to decrease levels of HIV when patients are treated with acyclovir for genital herpes.

Herpes Simplex Encephalitis

In rare cases, as with infants, herpes viruses can enter the brains of adolescents and adults and cause herpes simplex encephalitis. This potentially damaging and deadly disease accounts for 10 percent of all encephalitis cases—numbering in the hundreds to several thousand cases annually—although experts suspect that the number is much higher since many cases go unrecognized. Herpes simplex encephalitis infection causes irritation and swelling of the brain tissues and sometimes brain hemorrhaging. Some people infected with herpes simplex encephalitis may only have mild, flu-like symptoms such as fever and headache. In extreme cases individuals can suffer brain damage, memory loss, partial paralysis, seizures, speech problems, or stroke.

Untreated herpes simplex encephalitis progresses rapidly and causes death within just one or two weeks in more than 50 percent of cases. According to the National Institute of Neurological Disorders and Stroke, "This rapidly progressing disease is the single most important cause of fatal sporadic encephalitis in the U.S. Brain damage in adults and in children beyond the neonatal period is usually seen in the frontal and temporal lobes and can be severe."[23] People most at risk for herpes simplex encephalitis are those who are undergoing chemotherapy or whose immune systems have been weakened by illnesses such as AIDS, diabetes, or Hodgkin's lymphoma.

Herpes of the Eye

Herpes infection of the eye, known as ocular herpes, is a common disease that has affected nearly a half-million American adults and children, with nearly 50,000 new and recurring cases each year. In 9 out of 10 cases, HSV-1, the virus responsible for oral herpes, infects only one eye. Experts do not completely understand why herpes simplex infects the eye in some people and not in others. Deborah Pavan Langston, an ophthalmologist at the Massachusetts Eye and Ear Infirmary in Boston, explains how ocular herpes develops:

> The source of infection is usually a family member or friend who is silently shedding virus in the saliva or nasal secretions, or who has an active cold sore. When the virus first enters the body, usually through the nose or mouth, it travels through the nerves up to the same center which also sends nerves to the eye. There it goes to sleep in an inactive infection state and may never reawaken. Occasionally, the virus does reactivate (stress!) and, instead of

traveling back down the nerves to the mouth or nose, it goes to the eye causing the illness there.[24]

Studies have shown that people who have an initial ocular herpes outbreak have up to a 50 percent chance of recurring infection.

Several types of ocular herpes can cause symptoms ranging from simple infections and redness in the eye to conditions that can lead to permanent blindness. Keratitis is the most common type of ocular herpes—generally affecting only the top layer of the cornea—causing symptoms such as pain, redness, sensitivity to light, and blurred vision. However, scarring of the eye may occur without prompt treatment with antiviral drugs or eyedrops. Stromal keratitis, accounting for 25 percent of ocular herpes, infects deeper layers of the cornea, may be more difficult to treat, and can lead to scarring, glaucoma, loss of vision, and blindness. Less commonly, herpes simplex may infect the inside of the eye (herpes uveitis) and the back of the eye (herpes retinitis). People infected with these two types of ocular herpes are at risk of cataracts, glaucoma, and retinal detachment, and permanent vision loss can result without treatment.

> " Herpes infection of the eye, known as ocular herpes, is a common disease that has affected nearly a half-million American adults and children, with nearly 50,000 new and recurring cases each year. "

Early Treatment Is Critical

Physicians and experts warn that certain individuals with herpes infections are at high risk of developing lasting or severe complications. Newborns, people who have undergone organ transplants, and others whose immune systems are weak or impaired could suffer damage to the central nervous system or develop pneumonia, hepatitis, or other illnesses. Doctors stress that getting early treatment via antiviral drugs or other means is critical for these at-risk individuals to keep their herpes infections in check.

What Are the Health Effects of Herpes?

Primary Source Quotes

66 **Though rare, contact with herpes sores during delivery can lead to a severe, life-threatening infection for the baby.** 99

—Planned Parenthood, "Herpes & Pregnancy," 2010. www.plannedparenthood.org.

Planned Parenthood is an organization that provides health care, sex education, and information to the public.

66 **A first herpes infection during pregnancy (especially the third trimester) poses a significant risk of infection of the fetus while in the womb as well as during delivery.** 99

—Elizabeth Stein, "Top Tips for Pregnant Women with Herpes Simplex Virus," EmpowHer, March 4, 2010. www.empowher.com.

Stein practices obstetrics and gynecology in New York City.

* Editor's Note: While the definition of a primary source can be narrowly or broadly defined, for the purposes of Compact Research, a primary source consists of: 1) results of original research presented by an organization or researcher; 2) eyewitness accounts of events, personal experience, or work experience; 3) first-person editorials offering pundits' opinions; 4) government officials presenting political plans and/or policies; 5) representatives of organizations presenting testimony or policy.

BBNewborns with herpes simplex virus skin disease have recurrences for months to years, particularly with HSV-2 disease, even if antiviral therapy was administered."

—Swetha G. Pinninti, "Herpes Simplex Virus Infection: Follow-Up," eMedicine, March 4, 2010. www.emedicine.medscape.com.

Pinninti is a pediatrician at St. Peter's University Hospital in New Brunswick, New Jersey.

BBPersons with HIV can have severe herpes outbreaks, and this may help facilitate transmission of both herpes and HIV infections to other persons."

—Illinois Department of Public Health, "Healthbeat: Genital Herpes," January 2008. www.idph.state.il.us.

The Illinois Department of Public Health is a state agency responsible for promoting and protecting public health.

BBHerpes simplex virus (HSV-2) coinfection is associated with increased plasma and genital-tract HIV RNA [genetic material] levels and may increase the risk for HIV transmission."

—Rajesh Gandhi, "HIV/HSV-2 Coinfection: Disappointing Results for Acyclovir Suppression," *Journal Watch*, January 20, 2010. www.jwatch.org.

Gandhi is the director of HIV Clinical Services and Education at Massachusetts General Hospital in Boston and an associate professor of medicine at Harvard University Medical School.

BBDespite advances in antiviral therapy over the past 2 decades, herpes simplex encephalitis (HSE) remains a serious illness with significant risks of morbidity and death."

—Todd Pritz, "Herpes Simplex Encephalitis," eMedicine, January 7, 2010. www.emedicine.medscape.com.

Pritz is a physician practicing internal medicine at St. Anthony's Medical Center in St. Louis, Missouri.

❝ Herpes of the eye, or ocular herpes, is a recurrent viral infection that is caused by the herpes simplex virus and is the most common infectious cause of corneal blindness in the U.S. **❞**

—National Eye Institute, "Facts About the Cornea and Corneal Disease," April 2010. www.nei.nih.gov.

The National Eye Institute in Bethesda, Maryland, is part of the National Institutes of Health.

....

❝ HSV can be life-threatening to a person who has cancer, an individual with AIDS, a person who has had an organ transplant, or anyone who has some other major illness, because their immunity to infection has been reduced. **❞**

—American Academy of Dermatology, "Herpes Simplex," 2010. www.aad.org.

The American Academy of Dermatology in Schaumburg, Illinois, represents virtually all practicing dermatologists in the United States.

....

❝ In some people whose immune systems do not work properly . . . genital herpes outbreaks can be unusually severe and long lasting. **❞**

—National Institute of Allergy and Infectious Diseases, "Genital Herpes: Complications," March 19, 2010. www.niaid.nih.gov.

The National Institute of Allergy and Infectious Diseases, an agency of the National Institutes of Health, conducts research on infectious, immunologic, and allergic diseases.

....

What Are the Health Effects of Herpes?

- It takes approximately **7 to 10 days** for skin to return to normal after herpes sores appear.

- According to the National Institute of Allergic and Infectious Diseases, in the United States approximately **1,500 babies** are born with herpes each year.

- Neonatal herpes can cause **birth defects, low birth weight**, and **death** in afflicted infants.

- **Infants** may acquire oral herpes if their skin is touched after birth by an infected adult.

- People who have both the **herpes and HIV viruses** are more likely to transmit either disease to their sexual partners.

- **Open sores or breaks** in the skin caused by herpes viruses can be a way for HIV to enter the body.

- **AIDS** may develop more quickly in people infected with both genital herpes and HIV.

- **Herpes simplex encephalitis** can cause mild, flu-like symptoms but also brain damage and death.

How Herpes Sores Develop

Oral and genital herpes are common and highly infectious. Both are caused by the herpes simplex virus, which results in painful blisters and sores on the skin around the mouth or genitals.

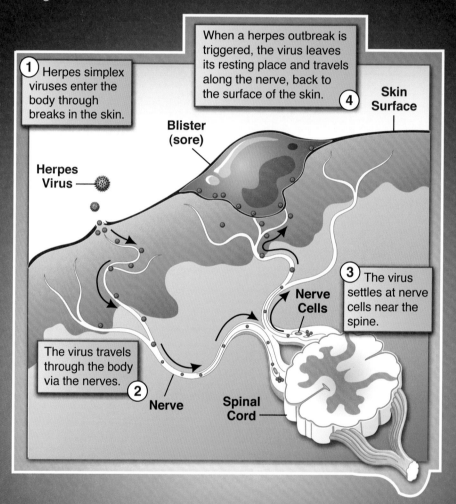

1 Herpes simplex viruses enter the body through breaks in the skin.

When a herpes outbreak is triggered, the virus leaves its resting place and travels along the nerve, back to the surface of the skin. 4

Skin Surface

Blister (sore)

Herpes Virus

3 The virus settles at nerve cells near the spine.

Nerve Cells

The virus travels through the body via the nerves.

2 **Nerve**

Spinal Cord

Source: American Congress of Obstetricians and Gynecologists, "Genital Herpes," pamphlet, 2008. www.acog.org.

- Herpes simplex is responsible for about **10 percent** of the 20,000 cases of encephalitis that occur annually in the United States.

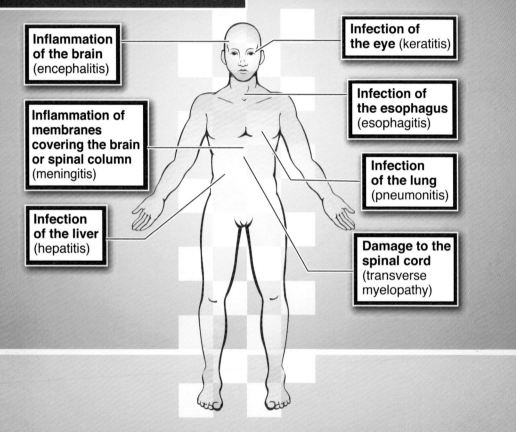

Diseases Associated with Disseminated Herpes Infection

People with weakened immune systems, pregnant women, and newborns are considered at risk for what is known as disseminated herpes infection. This infection is characterized by organ failure in one or more parts of the body.

Inflammation of the brain (encephalitis)

Infection of the eye (keratitis)

Inflammation of membranes covering the brain or spinal column (meningitis)

Infection of the esophagus (esophagitis)

Infection of the liver (hepatitis)

Infection of the lung (pneumonitis)

Damage to the spinal cord (transverse myelopathy)

Source: Monica Gandhi, "Genital Herpes," Knol, October 28, 2008. http://knol.google.com.

- The National Eye Institute estimates that **400,000** Americans have had some form of ocular herpes.

Pregnant Women and STDs

Of all STDs, genital herpes is the most common among pregnant women. This is a concern because women infected with genital herpes are at risk for passing on the virus to their babies during pregnancy and delivery. Infection of the fetus or newborn can result in serious health problems affecting the brain, eyes, lungs, and gastrointestinal tract. The graph shows the annual estimated number of pregnant women with STDs in the United States.

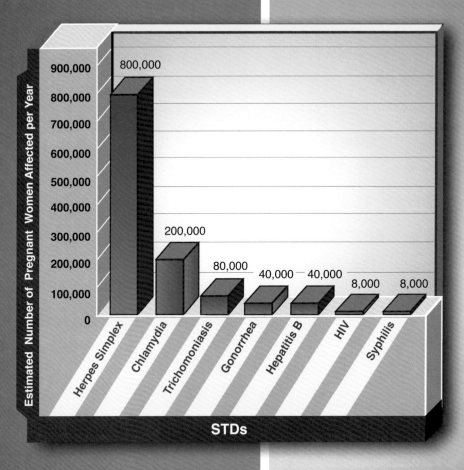

Source: Centers for Disease Control and Prevention, "STDs and Pregnancy," December 2007. www.cdc.gov.

How Can Herpes Be Treated?

66Antiviral drugs, such as acyclovir and more recently, valacyclovir and famciclovir, have been known to reduce herpes outbreaks for nearly two decades.99

—Fred Hutchinson Cancer Research Center, a medical facility in Seattle, Washington.

66There are natural treatment options that can be very effective in reducing the length and severity of outbreaks.99

—Sheldon Miller, a health researcher who has studied natural remedies for herpes and other STDs.

I n 1974 biochemist Gertrude Elion began to study a chemical compound called acyclovir that had just been created at her pharmaceutical company based in North Carolina. Elion had won acclaim 20 years earlier by creating the first drug treatment for acute childhood leukemia. Her research strategy was that infectious diseases could be fought if drugs could be targeted to attack bacterial and viral DNA. Elion and her team began studying how acyclovir worked, why it worked, and why it was not toxic to normal cells. They discovered that acyclovir remains inactive until it comes into contact with herpes viruses. The drug then interferes with the enzymes these viruses need to reproduce in the body. In 1982 acyclovir was approved by the U.S. Food and Drug Administration (FDA) as the first drug to treat herpes infections. In 1988 Elion shared the Nobel Prize in Physiology or Medicine for her important discoveries in drug research.

Acyclovir and its related drugs—famciclovir and valacyclovir—are the only drugs approved by the FDA to treat herpes infections. Famciclovir and valacyclovir became available by prescription in 1996. Today each of these drugs—both in generic and brand-name form—are available at pharmacies or on the Internet with or without a doctor's prescription, and they are exceedingly safe to use, with no damaging side effects. These antivirals work in similar fashion: Primarily taken orally, they reduce the pain and frequency of outbreaks, help herpes sores heal faster, and reduce the amount of HSV-2 that is shed from the genital area, which is the major source of herpes transmission.

> **While the three drugs are equally effective at suppressing recurrences, valacyclovir helps prevent the transmission of genital herpes, a benefit not duplicated in clinical trials with the other two drugs.**

While the three drugs are equally effective at suppressing recurrences, valacyclovir helps prevent the transmission of genital herpes, a benefit not duplicated in clinical trials with the other two drugs. In 2004 an international research team led by Lawrence Corey of the Fred Hutchinson Cancer Research Center found that taking a daily dose of valacyclovir reduced the transmission of genital herpes to uninfected partners by 50 percent. According to Corey, head of the center's infectious diseases program: "This is the first demonstration that an antiviral drug can prevent a viral sexually transmitted disease. The study provides the conceptual framework to extend the approach to other viral sexually transmitted diseases, such as HIV infection."[25]

How the Drugs Act in the Body

Although the introduction of acyclovir broke new ground in the world of medicine, the drug had one significant drawback: Taken orally, only 15 to 20 percent of the medicine is absorbed by the body and available for use. In other words, acyclovir "washes out" of the body very quickly. Therefore, the drug needs to be taken often each day—usually two to three times daily—to remain effective against herpes. Still, it is the most widely prescribed and the least costly of the three medicines. Conversely, famciclovir and valacyclovir are both well absorbed. The body utilizes a much higher percentage of these drugs, so they require less frequent dosing.

Once inside the body, antiviral drugs play a trick on the herpes virus. As researcher Terri Warren notes, "These medicines present themselves to the virus as one of the nutrients it needs, but they're really just pretenders. When the virus takes up the pretender medicine to make more DNA to reproduce, it can't do it, because the look-alike nutrient isn't the real thing."[26] Although the virus is not completely eliminated from the body, its replication is thwarted so that outbreaks and shedding are reduced.

Any of the three antiviral drugs can be taken to combat first-episode outbreaks. The key is receiving treatment early enough so that the virus does not disseminate and proceed to cause painful symptoms. During initial genital herpes outbreaks, the medicines are taken over a 7- to 10-day period and can shorten the duration of herpes symptoms by 40 to 50 percent. Some people with first episodes may at first have mild symptoms but then experience new sores shortly thereafter. Antiviral medications can prevent this second round of sores from occurring.

Choice of Therapies

Most people with genital herpes have four to six outbreaks in the first year that they have the virus. Antiviral drugs are just as effective for recurring episodes. After initial episodes, individuals have a choice of pursuing episodic therapy or suppressive therapy after consulting their physician.

Episodic therapy is a regimen in which medicine is taken for several days only during an outbreak. This type of treatment is most effective when it begins at the first warning sign, such as itching or tingling. In many cases, if treatment begins early enough, the outbreak will end before herpes sores appear. Episodic treatment shortens the duration of symptoms and speeds the healing of sores, but it

> **The key is receiving treatment early enough so that the virus does not disseminate and proceed to cause painful symptoms.**

does not reduce the frequency of outbreaks. It is generally used by people who have few outbreaks or mild symptoms.

> **Episodic treatment shortens the duration of symptoms and speeds the healing of sores, but it does not reduce the frequency of outbreaks.**

Suppressive therapy involves taking medication every day, whether someone is having an outbreak or not. It is the approach usually recommended for individuals who have frequent (six or more) outbreaks per year. In order to reduce the chance of recurrences or avoid them altogether, patients can take a small dose of antiviral medication every day for long periods of time, sometimes for up to three years. The main goal of suppressive therapy is to reduce the number of recurrences each year and to improve quality of life. If an outbreak occurs during suppressive therapy, the healing time is short, with less severe symptoms. Once herpes outbreaks are reduced, physicians may gradually decrease the dose of the antiviral drug.

Relief for Oral Herpes

Acyclovir, famciclovir, and valacyclovir are all FDA-approved oral medications for the treatment of oral herpes too. In addition, there are many other topical creams and ointments that may reduce pain, heal sores faster, or do both. Some creams contain a small amount of an antiviral agent. Acyclovir cream, for example, contains 5 percent acyclovir and is commonly prescribed for oral herpes. It requires frequent application, every two hours for several days. Penciclovir is an antiviral medication that, because it is poorly absorbed by the body, is more effective against oral herpes when used in topical cream. Docosanol cream is the only FDA-approved nonprescription ointment for oral herpes and is applied five times per day. Several other over-the-counter topical anesthetics in the form of creams or lotions—such as lidocaine—can also provide relief. Many people also rely on aspirin, acetaminophen, or ibuprofen to reduce fever, aches, and inflammation associated with herpes.

Controversial Treatments

Much has been written and advertised about quick or immediate relief for herpes. Numerous Web sites, for example, tout their products as effective treatments with guaranteed results, some even citing them as "breakthroughs" or "cures." Many health experts warn that such Web sites are filled with misinformation and exaggeration and that these unconventional and unproven products should be avoided. These skeptics add that products marketed without rigorous testing may work for one person but just as likely may not work for another.

One such controversial product is dimethyl sulfoxide (DMSO), an over-the-counter skin-penetrating solvent that has been approved by the FDA for only one medical purpose: to relieve pain from a rare bladder disorder. Warnings about using DMSO to treat herpes date back to the 1980s. For many years consumers have purchased DMSO as a cream not only to treat herpes, but for other conditions, including arthritis relief, sexual dysfunction, and sports injuries. But in the words of author Christopher Scipio, an herbalist who writes frequently about herpes treatments: "DMSO has never been shown to be an effective therapy for the treatment of herpes either in peer-reviewed clinical studies or in clinical practice by those treating herpes. In my 16 years of treating herpes I have never met or heard of any herpes treatment specialist advocating the use of . . . DMSO."[27]

> " From aloe vera to zinc, dozens of vitamins, herbs, extracts, and minerals are available to treat oral and genital herpes. "

In addition to DMSO, there are many other tablets, creams, and liquids on the market with catchy brand names promising quick relief to people with herpes. According to Elizabeth Boskey, a researcher who has written books and articles on sexual health, "I have read many posts from people desperately hoping for a herpes cure; these are people who look for any evidence at all that the claims could be true, while ignoring any evidence that it is not."[28]

Boskey and others note that many product Web sites deceive consumers by claiming a quick fix for herpes but then qualifying these claims with printed text—often in small print—that no cure exists for herpes. Boskey adds, "Treatments that are misleadingly advertised as herpes cures may encourage individuals to make dangerous decisions about safe sex because they believe that their partners are no longer at risk."[29] Experts suggest that consumers do their own research to avoid falling prey to misleading and deceptive advertising, focusing on remedies that have been adequately tested and recommended, if not by physicians, then by others with herpes who have found products to be successful.

A Natural Approach

Many people with herpes seek relief by using natural alternatives instead of traditional medicine. From aloe vera to zinc, dozens of vitamins, herbs, extracts, and minerals are available to treat oral and genital herpes. These remedies come in many forms, such as capsules, pills, liquids, creams, lotions, and powders and are either ingested or used directly on sores. According to natural health practitioners, such natural remedies may be beneficial by healing sores, preventing herpes viruses from replicating, and strengthening the immune system to prevent outbreaks. For example, some studies have shown that herbs, vitamins, and minerals such as echinacea, vitamin C, and zinc can boost the body's immune system by increasing production of and strengthening lymphocytes and other white blood cells, which are important bodily defenses against viral infections. As Susan Kowalsky, a naturopathic doctor in Vermont, writes, "It's known that viruses deplete vitamin C residing in white blood cells, so we know that if you want your immune system to stay strong, you need to take extra vitamin C."[30]

These natural defenses are an important tool in fighting off herpes outbreaks and are one part of maintaining a well-balanced diet and healthy lifestyle. According to Jared Hanson, a naturopathic physician in New York City:

> The first goal of natural treatment for herpes is to support the immune system, which is responsible for keeping the virus in check. Optimizing immune response requires certain lifestyle and dietary adjustments as well as supplementation with key immune nutrients. . . . A host of vitamins, minerals and other nutrients are necessary for the immune system. Vitamins A, C, D and E as well as the B vitamins are important, as well as the minerals iron, selenium and zinc.[31]

In addition to practicing a healthy lifestyle, people with herpes can benefit from simple and immediate techniques, such as placing ice packs on sores, bathing in salt water or therapeutic baths, wearing loose clothing, or avoiding sunlight. Using small amounts of bleach, hydrogen peroxide, and iodine as drying agents on sores has also been recommended by people with herpes, some of whom claim that rubbing ear wax on oral herpes sores also helps them heal quickly.

Hope, Not Despair

Regardless of whether people treat their herpes infections with traditional medicines or natural remedies, prompt and adequate care and treatment can mean a tremendous difference in living as normal a lifestyle as possible, protecting one's sexual partners, and avoiding burdensome pain and discomfort. Beyond the initial emotional and physical distress felt when people learn that they have contracted herpes, today this very common disease can become quite manageable. With increasing medical and educational resources available, herpes need not be viewed as a dire, hopeless condition by those who have it.

How Can Herpes Be Treated?

66 It turns out that we have really good drugs that kill productively replicating herpes simplex viruses that are approved drugs that are commercially available. 99

—Bryan Cullen, National Public Radio interview, July 2, 2008.

Cullen is a molecular genetics professor at Duke University in North Carolina.

66 Studies show that the side effects and risks of daily antiviral therapy are no more common than in people who take intermittent antivirals for herpes outbreaks. 99

—Charlotte Grayson, "Five Questions to Ask Your Doctor About Suppressive Therapy," February 20, 2009.
www.healthcentral.com.

Grayson practices internal medicine in Fayetteville, Georgia.

* Editor's Note: While the definition of a primary source can be narrowly or broadly defined, for the purposes of Compact Research, a primary source consists of: 1) results of original research presented by an organization or researcher; 2) eyewitness accounts of events, personal experience, or work experience; 3) first-person editorials offering pundits' opinions; 4) government officials presenting political plans and/or policies; 5) representatives of organizations presenting testimony or policy.

66 The bottom line for most people is that herpes is simply an occasional physical annoyance that can be treated with medication.**99**

—Lisa Marr, *Sexually Transmitted Diseases: A Physician Tells You What You Need to Know*. Baltimore, MD: Johns Hopkins University Press, 2007.

Marr practices geriatric medicine in Milwaukee, Wisconsin.

....

66 By treating the infected partner with suppressive therapy, transmission of symptomatic herpes can be prevented in over 90 percent of cases.**99**

—Johns Hopkins Bayview Medical Center, "Herpes FAQs," 2008. www.hopkinsbayview.org.

Founded in 1773, the Johns Hopkins Bayview Medical Center is a full-service academic medical center located in Baltimore, Maryland.

....

66 For some, nonprescription pain medications like aspirin, acetaminophen, or ibuprofen can alleviate the pain and discomfort caused by the sores.**99**

—Lawrence R. Stanberry, *Understanding Herpes*. Jackson: University Press of Mississippi, 2006.

Stanberry is a prominent herpes researcher and author.

....

66 Over-the-counter creams and/or ointments are not recommended for genital herpes, since they can interfere with the healing process in a number of ways, causing genital outbreaks to last longer. Keeping the area clean and as dry as possible and allowing the area to get air can help to speed the healing process.**99**

—American Social Health Association, "Learn About Herpes," 2010. www.ashastd.org.

The American Social Health Association is a nonprofit public health organization in North Carolina.

....

66 Just because doctors and scientists don't have enough conclusive evidence to make a general recommendation about lysine doesn't mean it might not be a good adjunct herpes treatment in some people. 99

—Elizabeth Boskey, "Is Lysine an Effective Treatment for Herpes?" About.com, August 31, 2009. http://std.about.com.

Boskey is a researcher, writer, and educator on the subject of STDs.

66 The problem with alternative treatments is that large studies haven't been done to prove whether or not they really work. 99

—Terri Warren, *The Good News About the Bad News: Herpes; Everything You Need to Know*. Oakland, CA: New Harbinger, 2009.

Warren operates the Westover Heights Clinic in Portland, Oregon, a private clinic specializing in the diagnosis and treatment of sexually transmitted diseases.

How Can Herpes Be Treated?

- HSV-1 and HSV-2 are very similar viruses that share about **50 percent** of the same genes.

- The Federal Trade Commission and the U.S. Food and Drug Administration monitor companies that advertise herpes treatments and have **penalized those touting a cure**.

- **Acyclovir** was the first drug approved by the U.S. Food and Drug Administration to treat herpes.

- Physicians have successfully treated some infants with herpes with **high daily doses** of acyclovir for two to three weeks.

- Valacyclovir is an antiviral drug commonly known by its brand name, **Valtrex**.

- A five-year study led by the University of Washington in Seattle found that acyclovir, a drug used to suppress the symptoms of herpes, **did not reduce HIV transmission** by people with both viruses.

- Episodic treatment of herpes **does not reduce the recurrence** of outbreaks.

- **Recurrent genital herpes** is most common in the first year after the initial infection and decreases as time goes on.

Possible Side Effects of Antiviral Drugs

Antiviral drugs have been effective in reducing the duration and frequency of herpes outbreaks for many people. As with any drug, however, antivirals may also have unwanted side effects and certain people—pregnant women, for instance—may find the effects particularly problematic.

Drug	Potential Side Effects	May Cause Problems For
acyclovir (Zovirax)	stomach upset; loss of appetite; nausea; vomiting; diarrhea; headache dizziness; weakness	people with kidney disease; pregnant or nursing women
famciclovir (Famvir)	nausea; diarrhea; headache; fatigue	people with kidney disease; pregnant or nursing women
valacyclovir (Valtrex)	nausea; vomiting; headache; loss of appetite; weakness; stomach pain; dizziness	people with kidney disease; pregnant or nursing women; the elderly

Source: WebMD, "Genital Herpes Medications Chart," 2010. www.webmd.com.

- Estimated direct costs of treating HSV-2 in the United States alone are close to **$1 billion** annually, primarily for drugs and outpatient medical care.

- One study of 115 patients with oral herpes lip sores showed significant improvement in those who used a topical cream containing **lemon balm extract** compared with patients who used a placebo cream.

Most Common Herpes Symptoms and Treatments

A survey conducted by the herpes information Web site herpes.com suggests that the number of people using prescription medications for herpes is almost equal to the number of people who use no treatment of any kind. Vitamins and herbs and stress reduction techniques are the next most common forms of treatment for herpes, according to the survey (which involved more than 40,000 people who also addressed questions about symptoms, duration, and frequency of outbreaks).

Symptoms Experienced During Lesion Formation	
Sharp pain:	39.3%
Muscle aches:	36.2%
Swollen lymph glands:	34.3%
Headaches:	32%
Fever and/or general malaise	27.9%
Treatment	
Prescription:	27.5%
Over-the-counter treatment:	4.7%
Psychotherapy:	1.3%
Diet and nutrition:	16%
Vitamins and herbs:	18.8%
Stress reduction:	17.5%
No treatment:	27.9%
Frequency of Outbreak Recurrences	
1 time from 1–5 years:	40.7%
4–7 times per year:	38.7%
1–2 times per month:	20.6%
Average Duration of Outbreaks	
1–3 days duration:	19.6%
4–7 days duration:	45.8%
8–10 days duration:	17.7%
More than 10 days duration:	16.8%

How Can the Spread of Herpes Be Prevented?

> **The primary aim of a public health approach to preventing HSV transmission is to reduce transmission to uninfected partners.**
>
> —Cornelis A. Rietmeijer, a physician with the Denver Public Health Department in Colorado.

> **At present, our national strategy to control HSV-2 is not well defined, nor have we made a commitment to developing a national strategy.**
>
> —Matthew Golden, a University of Washington associate professor of medicine.

When Angela, a 25-year-old from Omaha, Nebraska, underwent treatment for a suspected bladder infection, she began experiencing severe pain and could not walk. After insisting on a vaginal examination, Angela learned that she in fact had genital herpes. She realized she had contracted the virus from a sexual contact just weeks earlier. Prior to having sex, neither she nor her partner had discussed having any sexually transmitted diseases, and she was angry that her partner had not informed her that he had herpes. After receiving a prescription for antiviral medications, Angela set out to learn more about her disease.

With increased knowledge about herpes, Angela decided that the best course of action was to stay on her medication and to inform the men she dated about her infection. Over the next two years, she took her pills daily and managed to stay outbreak free. She also organized her own local herpes support group. When Angela began dating her future husband, she was apprehensive about telling him that she had genital herpes, but was relieved when he reacted supportively. Angela decided to stop taking her herpes medications, except during the latter weeks of her two pregnancies, and has gone years without any outbreaks. Angela writes: "Telling a potential partner that you have herpes is not always easy but I think we can agree it's the right thing to do. My advice to anybody that is newly diagnosed would be to educate yourself as much as possible."[32] Many doctors stress that the proactive approach taken by Angela and people like her is vital in helping to prevent the spread of genital herpes.

Efforts to Stem a Serious Threat

According to a CDC survey conducted between 1988 and 1994, of 40,000 Americans tested, 20.8 percent were found to be infected with genital herpes. Similar studies later found that this percentage had dropped to 17 percent by 2004 and to 16 percent by 2008. Despite this progress, researchers note that approximately 1 million new infections occur every year, which means that public awareness must still be raised and prevention strategies must be put in place to further reduce the spread of herpes.

Commenting in March 2010 on the latest survey, Kevin Fenton, a CDC director, says: "This study serves as a stark reminder that herpes remains a common and serious health threat in the United States. Everyone should be aware of the symptoms, risk factors, and steps that can be taken to prevent the spread of this lifelong and incurable infection."[33] Experts argue that multipronged strategies, from personal choices of determining when and with whom to have sex to large-scale public education efforts, are required to keep uninfected people free from herpes.

> " Researchers note that public awareness must still be raised and prevention strategies must be put in place to further reduce the spread of herpes. "

Limiting Sexual Activity

It is a common warning that the only sure ways to avoid genital herpes infections are to abstain from sexual contact altogether or to be in a monogamous relationship with a person who has been tested and found not to have herpes. Under other circumstances, it is important for people to consider when *not* to have sex. Public health organizations advise against any sexual contact when someone has visible herpes sores or is experiencing symptoms such as tingling. Other steps include limiting one's number of sexual partners and avoiding sex with someone who may already have herpes or other STDs. According to the Minnesota Department of Health: "As with other STDs, your sexual habits and patterns determine the likelihood of being exposed and infected. The more frequently a person engages in sexual relations with different people, the greater the risk of acquiring genital herpes or another STD. Limiting the number of sexual partners will greatly improve your chances of avoiding genital herpes."[34]

> **Millions of people rely on condoms as a precautionary measure to reduce the risk of transmitting or contracting herpes and other STDs.**

Other experts may agree, but they contend that other factors must be considered. In the words of author and sex therapist Ruth Westheimer: "Some people with herpes got it because they were promiscuous, but most weren't. One could say that for the latter group it was mostly a case of bad luck, but with herpes being so widespread, the odds of getting it aren't all that low."[35]

Testing for Herpes

An important strategy that may help prevent the spread of herpes involves getting tested for the disease, according to many health experts. Their hope is that if people discover they are infected with herpes, they will take certain steps—such as using condoms or abstaining from sex when they know they are contagious—to prevent exposing others to the disease. People who suspect they may have genital herpes can get one of several types of tests administered by a physician. The most common test is known as a culture test, in which a doctor swabs a lesion for a sample to be tested in a lab. Culture tests, however, often produce "false negatives," meaning that the test does not detect herpes when in fact the person actually is infected.

Another test is a blood test, also known as a serologic test. Blood tests do not detect the presence of the herpes virus. Instead, they detect certain antibodies (the body's immune response to the virus) in the blood. One advantage of the blood test is that it can still let patients know if they have herpes long after symptoms have disappeared. One very accurate test is the polymerase chain reaction (PCR) test, which detects the genetic material of herpes viruses. The PCR test can identify whether a person is infected with HSV-1 or HSV-2; however, because of the higher cost it is not as widely available as culture tests or blood tests.

Condoms and Herpes

Millions of people rely on condoms as a precautionary measure to reduce the risk of transmitting or contracting herpes and other STDs. A study published in the *Archives of Internal Medicine* in July 2009 found that consistent condom users have approximately a 30 percent lower risk of contracting genital herpes than those who never use condoms. According to Emily T. Martin, the study's lead researcher, "Thirty percent is partial protection, but it is protection."[36] Martin and other experts caution, however, that despite the increased protection from condoms, the risk of herpes infection is not entirely eliminated, because condoms leave areas of skin exposed where the virus may be present. As the authors of the Web site Herpes Diagnosis write:

> Because of the risk of transmission from subclinical shedding, it is helpful to use condoms for penetrative sex in between outbreaks. Condoms restrict contact between the penis and the mucosal surfaces of the vagina, mouth or anus, where subclinical shedding is known to occur. Be advised: Condoms may not cover all sites of viral shedding, and they don't provide a 100% guarantee against herpes transmission. For example, herpes sores may be present on the scrotum or upper thigh, or virus may be shed into vaginal secretions that would reach places not covered.[37]

Besides condoms worn by males, other products may be useful to avoid herpes infection. The female condom is a thin, lubricated sheath made of synthetic material. At one end is a closed inner ring that is inserted into the vagina to keep the condom in place. An outer ring at the opposite end is open and stays outside the vagina. Another product is known as the dental dam, a square piece of latex that a female uses to cover the vaginal area while receiving oral sex. This provides a barrier to the mouth of the other partner so that both skin contact and the exchange of bodily fluids may be avoided. Female condoms and dental dams may offer protection to sexual partners, but as with male condoms, individuals could possibly be exposed to areas of herpes-infected skin that these products leave uncovered.

Promise Seen in Microbicides

Microbicides are chemical compounds that kill viruses and bacteria and are used in many types of soaps, for example. Since the early 1990s dozens of pharmaceutical companies worldwide have pursued the development of microbicides to prevent infection from herpes, HIV, and other STDs. These self-administered microbicides take many different forms: gels, creams, foams, suppositories, films, lubricants, sponges, or vaginal rings that slowly release the active ingredient. When applied to the vagina or rectum, microbicides aim to prevent infection from herpes in different ways. Some kill or immobilize viruses, preventing them from taking hold after entering the body. Others block infection by creating a barrier between viruses and skin cells, acting much like a "chemical condom."

> **Since the early 1990s dozens of pharmaceutical companies worldwide have pursued the development of microbicides to prevent infection from herpes, HIV, and other STDs.**

Although studies have found certain herpes microbicides to be effective in animal testing and initial, small-scale testing on women, the results of broader testing on females have not been as successful as researchers had hoped. But even though these microbicides have been deemed ineffective, scientists have garnered valuable knowledge and experience, which they can then devote to newer compounds being developed.

One genital herpes microbicide, developed by researchers at Harvard Medical School and Albert Einstein College of Medicine, has taken a unique approach compared with previous microbicides. Their strategy uses RNA interference, a mechanism that cells use to protect their genetic machinery from viruses and other threats. This technique employs what are called small interfering RNA molecules, or siRNAs, to inactivate two genes. One siRNA targets a gene of the herpes virus, thus preventing it from replicating. The other siRNA prevents a protein used by the virus from attaching to skin cells. This microbicide, tested so far on mice only, protected them from lethal doses of herpes.

> " Ideally, a successful vaccine would protect uninfected people from genital herpes under any circumstances. "

Perhaps the most promising finding of the study was that the microbicide protected against herpes infection for a full week after application. In the words of lead investigator Judy Lieberman, a Harvard pediatrics professor: "One of the attractive features of the compound we developed is that it creates in the tissue a state that's resistant to infection, even if applied up to a week before sexual exposure. This aspect has a real practicality to it. If we can reproduce these results in people, this could have a powerful impact on preventing transmission."[38] Although this particular microbicide had not been scheduled for human testing as of 2010, it is symbolic of efforts by many companies and organizations worldwide, such as the World Health Organization, to address the demand for a safe and effective microbicide against herpes and other STDs.

The Search for a Successful Vaccine

Even more than microbicides, research of herpes vaccines has gone on for more than two decades, with many millions of dollars spent on vaccine development. Ideally, a successful vaccine would protect uninfected people from genital herpes under any circumstances. Since the 1980s herpes vaccines have been available in some European countries. Despite much debate as to how effective these vaccines are, they have not been authorized for use in the United States.

The first major trial of a preventive vaccine in the United States was conducted by the pharmaceutical company GlaxoSmithKline and the National Institutes of Health. Beginning in 2003, it tracked more than 7,000 women ages 18 to 30. Earlier studies of the vaccine, Herpevac, had shown promise, but only among women uninfected with either of the 2 herpes viruses. Their risk of contracting genital herpes and developing symptoms was reduced by about 75 percent. However, Herpevac was not effective for women who already had HSV-1 or for any men. One major complaint of the vaccine was that because most people acquire HSV-1 by the time they are in their teens, the likeliest recipients would be preteen girls. Results of the multiyear study were expected in the near future.

In March 2010 a Massachusetts company, BioVex, announced it had begun small-scale testing in London, England, of its ImmunoVex vaccine. Similar to vaccines for measles, mumps, and polio, this vaccine uses live but harmless viruses. The herpes viruses involved have had specific genes removed so that they can neither cause disease nor escape the effects of the immune system. According to BioVex, its vaccine has been adequately tested and has been found to prevent herpes completely, suggesting that it may be more potent than previous vaccines.

On the Horizon

While drugs and treatments are available to control the symptoms of herpes, some being very effective and others amounting to nothing more than hype, none yet can prevent herpes infections. Many researchers predict that a successful microbicide or vaccine against herpes will emerge in the next 5 to 10 years. Considering there are more than 1 million new cases of genital herpes occurring each year in the United States alone—and many millions more worldwide—a weapon that stopped herpes would be a milestone discovery in the world of medicine and a welcome breakthrough that has been eagerly awaited for decades.

How Can the Spread of Herpes Be Prevented?

66 **I encourage everyone to consider lowering the risk by avoiding intimate contact during any possible symptom of the virus being active (itching, tingling, burning, or numb sensations anywhere below the waist).** 99

—Christopher Scipio, "How Easy Is It to Get Herpes from Oral Sex?" Wellsphere, August 24, 2008. www.wellsphere.com.

Scipio is a holistic practitioner who writes about herpes treatments.

66 **You will not get herpes if you only have sex with a monogamous partner who is not infected with herpes.** 99

—Lucy Boyd, "Herpes Prevention Methods," Livestrong.com, April 17, 2010. www.livestrong.com.

Boyd is a registered nurse and the author of two medical books.

* Editor's Note: While the definition of a primary source can be narrowly or broadly defined, for the purposes of Compact Research, a primary source consists of: 1) results of original research presented by an organization or researcher; 2) eyewitness accounts of events, personal experience, or work experience; 3) first-person editorials offering pundits' opinions; 4) government officials presenting political plans and/or policies; 5) representatives of organizations presenting testimony or policy.

66The more sex partners you have, the more likely you are to have herpes.99

—Terri Warren, *The Good News About the Bad News: Herpes; Everything You Need to Know*. Oakland, CA: New Harbinger, 2009.

Warren operates the Westover Heights Clinic in Portland, Oregon, a private clinic specializing in the diagnosis and treatment of sexually transmitted diseases.

66Correct and consistent use of latex condoms can reduce the risk of genital herpes.99

—Centers for Disease Control and Prevention, "Genital Herpes—CDC Fact Sheet," March 3, 2010. www.cdc.gov.

The Centers for Disease Control and Prevention is a federal agency that works to protect public health and safety.

66Since a condom may not cover all infected areas, even correct and consistent use of latex condoms cannot guarantee protection from genital herpes.99

—Palo Alto Medical Foundation, "Types of STIs: Genital Herpes," 2010. www.pamf.org.

The Palo Alto Medical Foundation comprises a variety of medical centers in northern California.

66If you are having a herpes outbreak, you should not have any sexual contact until all sores have healed, the scabs have fallen off, and the skin is normal again.99

—Center for Young Women's Health, "Herpes," November 2, 2009. www.youngwomenshealth.org.

The Center for Young Women's Health is an educational resource center in Boston, Massachusetts.

66 The success of vaccines for chickenpox and shingles, which are caused by a herpes virus called varicella-zoster virus, suggests that vaccines may work for HSV-2. 99

—National Institute of Allergy and Infectious Diseases, "NIAID Researcher Seeks Effective Vaccine for Genital Herpes," April 7, 2009. www.niaid.nih.gov.

The National Institute of Allergy and Infectious Diseases is a federal agency that conducts and supports research on infectious and allergic diseases.

66 It is important that we promote steps to prevent the spread of genital herpes, not only because herpes is a lifelong and incurable infection but also because of the linkage between herpes and HIV infection. 99

—John M. Douglas Jr., "Herpes Infects One in Six in U.S.," *BusinessWeek*, March 9, 2010. www.businessweek.com.

Douglas is the director of the Centers for Disease Control and Prevention's division of sexually transmitted disease prevention.

Facts and Illustrations

How Can the Spread of Herpes Be Prevented?

- In the United States about **70 percent** of adults have been exposed to oral herpes by the age of 40.

- Early warning signs such as **tingling or itching** can alert people to treat potential herpes outbreaks.

- Experts advise that the only proven method of avoiding herpes infection is **abstaining** from sexual contact.

- According to Planned Parenthood, oral and genital herpes infections can be **diagnosed by testing the tissue or fluid taken** from sores.

- It can take many years and millions of dollars for a herpes drug or vaccine to be adequately tested and be subjected to **regulatory approval**.

- Some **herpes vaccines** have been tested using live herpes viruses that have been altered so that they are unable to cause infection.

- Laboratory studies have shown that latex **condoms** and **dental dams** provide an **impenetrable barrier** to particles the size of herpes viruses.

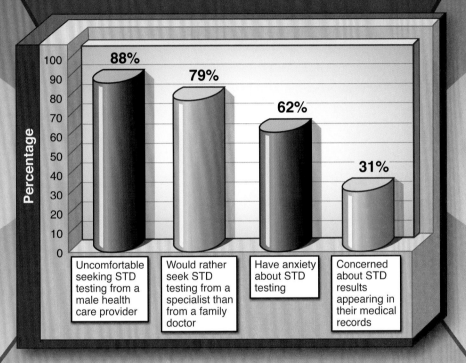

Barriers to STD Prevention and Treatment

One in 5 U.S. women, or 20 percent, are infected with genital herpes, according to the CDC. For African American women, the percentage is even higher, at 48 percent. Public health officials are concerned about the spread of herpes and other STDs among women. A survey of 302 women between the ages of 18 and 24 examined young women's beliefs about STD testing to find out why this important prevention tool is not used more often.

Source: Emma Hitt, "Young Women Face Barriers to STI Testing—Including Their Own Misconceptions," Medscape Medical News, March 18, 2010. www.medscape.com.

- According to the Global Campaign for Microbicides, dozens of products are being studied by scientists as potential **preventive microbicides** for sexually transmitted diseases, including herpes.

- In 2008 the World Health Organization estimated that **500 million people** worldwide were infected with genital herpes.

Stages of Drug Development

There are many stages involved in the creation, testing, and approval of drugs and medicines. Drugs, microbicides, and vaccines targeting herpes follow the same development pattern as other drugs, including rigorous testing on animals and people.

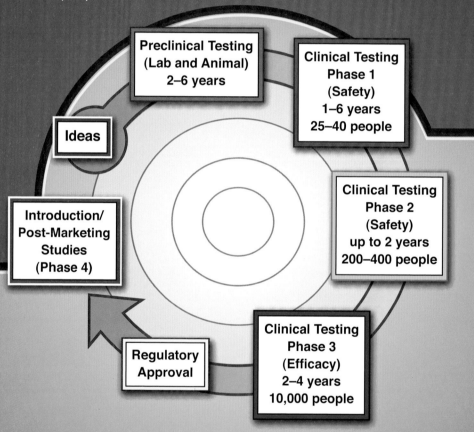

Preclinical Testing (Lab and Animal) 2–6 years

Clinical Testing Phase 1 (Safety) 1–6 years 25–40 people

Ideas

Clinical Testing Phase 2 (Safety) up to 2 years 200–400 people

Introduction/ Post-Marketing Studies (Phase 4)

Clinical Testing Phase 3 (Efficacy) 2–4 years 10,000 people

Regulatory Approval

Source: Global Campaign for Microbicides, "Testing & Trials," March 2007. www.global-campaign.org.

- A study of health clinics in Pittsburgh, Pennsylvania, found that women who treated **common vaginal infections** lowered their risk of contracting genital herpes.

- According to the Centers for Disease Control and Prevention, in the 1980s the number of clinically diagnosed cases of symptomatic genital herpes was **11 times greater than that in the 1970s**.

- Only a few U.S. states require that cases of genital herpes infections be **reported** to health authorities.

- According to health professionals, **proper nutrition, exercise, and rest** can help prevent genital herpes outbreaks.

- People infected with the genital herpes virus may **transmit** the virus even when they are not experiencing an outbreak.

Key People and Advocacy Groups

American Social Health Association: A national nonprofit organization that operates the Herpes Resource Center to provide the public with information about herpes.

Centers for Disease Control and Prevention: A federal agency that provides information to the public about diseases, including herpes, HIV, and other sexually transmitted diseases.

Lawrence Corey: A physician and scientist at the University of Washington in Seattle who is an internationally recognized expert on infectious diseases. Between 1988 and 1998 Corey published a series of key studies showing the association between infection with herpes simplex virus type 2 (HSV-2) and HIV.

International Herpes Management Forum: An organization established to improve the awareness and understanding of herpes viruses and the counseling and management of people with these infections.

National Institute of Allergy and Infectious Diseases: A federal agency that frequently partners with pharmaceutical companies to test herpes drugs such as microbicides and vaccines.

Lawrence Stanberry: The director of the Center for Vaccine Development at the University of Texas Medical Branch in Galveston. He has studied the development of herpes microbicides and vaccines, as well as the incidence of herpes among teens.

Vaccine and Infectious Disease Institute: Part of the Fred Hutchinson Cancer Research Center in Seattle, Washington. Its researchers have studied the transmission of herpes viruses and how herpes viruses act in the body.

Anna Wald: A professor of medicine and epidemiology at the University of Washington in Seattle who has taken part in many herpes studies. She is coauthor of the book *Managing Herpes: How to Live and Love with a Chronic STD.*

Terri Warren: The owner of Westover Heights Clinic in Portland, Oregon, a private clinic specializing in the diagnosis and treatment of sexually transmitted diseases. Warren is a national speaker and an author who has been involved in more than 100 clinical trials involving herpes testing, medications, and vaccines.

Chronology

1714
English physician Daniel Turner describes a herpes sore with yellow pus breaking through the skin.

1906
The term *herpes simplex* is introduced.

1893
French dermatologist Jean Baptiste Emile Vidal reports evidence that herpes is infectious.

1935
A case of neonatal herpes is reported for the first time by Harvard University pathologist George M. Hass.

1700

1900

1960

1736
French physician Jean Astruc publishes the first link between herpes and genital lesions in men and women.

1919
Scientist A. Lowenstein confirms experimentally the infectious nature of herpes simplex.

1886
The first book on the subject of genital herpes, *Les Herpes Genitaux*, is published in Paris, France.

1939
Medical researchers Frank M. Burnet and S.W. Williams theorize that herpes infections last for life.

1952
Microbiologist Cyril S. Stulberg and pediatrician Wolf W. Zuelzer describe eight fatal cases of generalized herpes simplex in newborn infants.

Chronology

1961
Scientists Karl E. Schneweis and Henning Brandis demonstrate the existence of two different types of herpes simplex virus: HSV-1 and HSV-2.

2010
Researchers announce the development of a microbicide that protects mice from lethal doses of herpes viruses.

1971
K.E. Schneweis of Bonn, Germany, and André Nahmias of Atlanta, Georgia, theorize that oral herpes and genital herpes are caused by two different types of herpes simplex virus.

1996
Antiviral herpes drugs famciclovir and valacyclovir become available by prescription.

1960

1985

2010

1964
Epstein-Barr virus, a disease-causing virus in the herpes virus family, is discovered by pathologist Michael Anthony Epstein.

2004
The Centers for Disease Control and Prevention reports that the prevalence of genital herpes in the United States decreased by 17 percent during the 1990s.

1979
New research suggests that herpes simplex may be a cause of Alzheimer's disease.

1990
A landmark paper by University of Washington researchers in the *Journal of the American Medical Association* shows that patients with genital herpes "shed" virus from the genital tract, even when they do not show any obvious symptoms.

1982
Acyclovir is approved for use as the first drug to treat herpes virus infections.

Related Organizations

Alice! Health Promotion Program at Columbia University

Wien Hall, Main Floor

411 W. 116th St.

New York, NY 10027

phone: (212) 854-5453 • fax: (212) 854-8949

e-mail: alice@columbia.edu • Web site: www.goaskalice.columbia.edu

This program at Columbia University helps students access information and resources, cultivates healthy attitudes and behaviors, and fosters a culture that values and supports a healthy community. It operates the Go Ask Alice! health question-and-answer Internet resource, which has an archive of herpes-related questions and answers.

American Academy of Dermatology (AAD)

PO Box 4014

Schaumburg, IL 60168

phone: (847) 330-0230; toll free: (866) 503-7546

fax: (847) 240-1859

Web site: www.aad.org

The AAD represents virtually all practicing dermatologists in the United States. It promotes leadership in dermatology and excellence in patient care through education, research, and advocacy. The AAD publishes pamphlets on herpes simplex and sexually transmitted diseases.

American Social Health Association (ASHA)

PO Box 13827

Research Triangle Park, NC 27709

phone: (919) 361-8400; toll free: (800) 227-8922 • fax: (919) 361-8425

e-mail: herpesnet@ashastd.org • Web site: www.ashastd.org

ASHA is a nonprofit organization that works to help improve public health. It sponsors the Herpes Resource Center to assist people with herpes. It publishes the *Helper* quarterly newsletter, the booklet *Understanding Herpes*, and the *Herpes Info Pack*. ASHA operates a telephone hotline and organizes help groups for people with herpes.

Center for Young Women's Health (CYWH)

333 Longwood Ave., 5th Floor

Boston, MA 02115

phone: (617) 355-2994 • fax: (617) 730-0186

Web site: www.youngwomenshealth.org

The CYWH provides education, clinical care, research, and health-care advocacy for teen girls and young women. Its online resources include numerous health guides for teens and parents, as well as information about sexually transmitted diseases, birth control, and general sexual health. It publishes the online quarterly newsletter *Teen Talk*.

Centers for Disease Control and Prevention (CDC)

Division of STD Prevention

1600 Clifton Rd.

Atlanta, GA 30333

phone: (800) 232-4636

e-mail: dstd@cdc.gov • Web site: www.cdc.gov/STD

The CDC's Division of STD Prevention helps people live safer, healthier lives by the prevention of STDs and their complications. Its Web site offers facts, statistics, and treatment information for genital herpes. Publications include fact sheets, which are also available in Spanish.

International Herpes Management Forum (IHMF)

IHMF Secretariat

Wicker House, High Street

Worthing, West Sussex, BN11 1DJ

United Kingdom

phone: (919) 361-8400; toll free: (800) 227-8922

fax: +44 (0)1903 520077

e-mail: ihmf@hbase.com • Web site: www.ihmf.com

Established in 1993, the IHMF is dedicated to improving the awareness, understanding, counseling, and management of herpes virus infections. Its review journal *Herpes* is published three times a year.

Mayo Clinic

200 First St. SW

Rochester, MN 55905

phone: (507) 284-2511; fax: (507) 284-0161

e-mail: dstd@cdc.gov • Web site: www.mayoclinic.com

The Mayo Clinic is a renowned not-for-profit medical practice and research group dedicated to the diagnosis and treatment of virtually every type of complex illness. The clinic employs more than 3,000 doctors, scientists, and health-care professionals. It publishes books on various health matters as well as the monthly newsletter *Mayo Clinic Health Letter*.

National Institute of Allergy and Infectious Diseases (NIAID)

6610 Rockledge Dr.

Bethesda, MD 20892-6612

phone: (301) 496-5717; toll free: (866) 284-4107 • fax: (301) 402-3573

e-mail: ocpostoffice@niaid.nih.gov • Web site: www.niaid.nih.gov

The NIAID conducts and supports research to help improve understanding, treatment, and prevention of infectious, immunologic, and allergic diseases. It publishes the monthly *NIH News in Health* newsletter.

Planned Parenthood

434 W. Thirty-third St.

New York, NY 10001

phone: (212) 541-7800; toll free: (800) 230-7526 • fax: (212) 245-1845

Web site: www.plannedparenthood.org

Planned Parenthood dates its beginnings to 1916, when Margaret Sanger helped open America's first birth control clinic in Brooklyn, New York. Since then it has expanded to more than 800 family planning and reproductive health centers across America which offer both STD testing and treatment.

Vaccine and Infectious Disease Institute (VIDI)

Fred Hutchinson Cancer Research Center

PO Box 19024, LE-500

Seattle, WA 98109

phone: (206) 667-4097 • fax: (206) 667-7711

Web site: www.fhcrc.org

VIDI was established by the Fred Hutchinson Cancer Research Center in 2007 to address the growing need for treatment and prevention strategies for infectious diseases worldwide. The institute has performed many studies on herpes transmission and vaccines. It publishes the monthly newsletter *VIDI Vitals.*

For Further Research

Books

Charles Ebel and Anna Wald, *Managing Herpes: Living and Loving with HSV*. Research Triangle Park, NC: American Social Health Association, 2007.

John W. Hill, *Natural Treatments for Genital Herpes, Cold Sores, and Shingles*. Yelm, WA: Clear Springs, 2008.

Adina Nack, *Damaged Goods? Women Living with Incurable Sexually Transmitted Diseases*. Philadelphia: Temple University Press, 2008.

Michele Picozzi, *Controlling Herpes Naturally: A Practical Guide to Treatment and Prevention*. 2nd ed. New Harmony, UT: Southpaw, 2006.

Christopher Scipio, *Making Peace with Herpes: A Holistic Guide to Overcoming the Stigma and Freeing Yourself from Outbreaks*. Sechelt, BC: Green Sun, 2008.

Lawrence R. Stanberry, *Understanding Herpes*. 2nd ed. Jackson: University Press of Mississippi, 2006.

Terri Warren, *The Good News About Bad News: Herpes; Everything You Need to Know*. Oakland, CA: New Harbinger, 2009.

Periodicals

Anonymous, "Commentary: Gambling with Herpes," *Essence*, March 11, 2010.

Centers for Disease Control and Prevention, "Sexually Transmitted Diseases Treatment Guidelines 2006," *Morbidity and Mortality Weekly Report*, August 4, 2006.

Lawrence Corey and Anna Wald, "Maternal and Neonatal Herpes Simplex Virus Infections," *New England Journal of Medicine*, October 1, 2009.

Boonsri Dickinson, "Harmful Herpes, Helpful Herpes," *Discover*, August 2007.

Martin Enserink, "Herpes Never Sleeps," *Science*, November 18, 2009.

Alexa Garcia-Ditta, "Herpes Healing Comes in Numbers," *Los Angeles Times*, January 11, 2010.

Carolyn Gardella, H. Hunter Handsfield, and Richard Whitley, "Neonatal Herpes—the Forgotten Perinatal Infection," *Sexually Transmitted Diseases*, January 2008.

Rachna Gupta, Anna Wald, and Terri Warren, "Genital Herpes," *Lancet*, December 22, 2007.

Edward W. Hook III, "An Evolving Understanding of Genital Herpes Pathogenesis: Is It Time for Our Approach to Therapy to Change as Well?" *Journal of Infectious Diseases*, January 20, 2010.

Laura Sanders, "How Herpes Re-Rears Its Ugly Head," *Science News*, April 25, 2009.

Mark R. Schleiss, "Cytomegalovirus Vaccines: At Last, a Major Step Forward," *Herpes*, vol. 15, no. 3, 2009.

ScienceDaily, "No More Cold Sores? Scientists Find Cellular Process That Fights Herpes Virus," March 24, 2009.

Jennifer Thomas, "Genital Herpes May Never Go Dormant," *HealthDay News*, November 18, 2009.

Aaron A.R. Tobian et al., "Male Circumcision for the Prevention of HSV-2 and HPV Infections and Syphilis," *New England Journal of Medicine*, March 26, 2009.

Internet Sources

Center for Young Women's Health, "Herpes," November 2009. www.youngwomenshealth.org/herpes.html.

Centers for Disease Control and Prevention, "Genital Herpes," November 2009. www.cdc.gov/std/herpes.

Female Symptoms Herpes and Signs, "Genital Herpes Symptoms," February 27, 2010. www.femalesymptomsherpes.net/category/uncategorized.

Herpes Coldsores Support Network, "Herpes—Sort the Facts from the Fiction," 2010. www.herpes-coldsores.com.

Herpes Doctor, "Public Forums," January 2010. www.herpesdoctor.com/forum.

Herpes.org, "February 2007 Newsletter," February 2007. www.herpes.org.

Herpesite, "Herpes and Relationships," 2010. www.herpesite.org/relationships.html.

Revolution Health, "Genital Herpes," February 5, 2008. www.revolutionhealth.com/conditions/stds/genital-herpes/index.

UpToDate, "What Is Genital Herpes?" January 22, 2009. www.utdol.com/patients/content/topic.do?topicKey=~25HoShXXwWUvwG.

Yoshi2me, "Herpes Help!" 2010. http://yoshi2me.com/herpes.

Source Notes

Overview

1. Holly Becker, "Herpes: My Story," Sex Etc., April 18, 2007. www.sexetc.org.
2. Becker, "Herpes."
3. Becker, "Herpes."
4. American Social Health Association, "Learn About Herpes," 2010. www.ashastd.org.
5. Melissa Conrad Stöppler, "Genital Herpes," eMedicineHealth, August 19, 2009. www.emedicinehealth.com.
6. Heather Brannon, "Genital Herpes Symptoms in Women," About.com, December 7, 2009. www.dermatology.about.com.
7. Centers for Disease Control and Prevention, "Genital Herpes—CDC Fact Sheet," March 3, 2010. www.cdc.gov.
8. American Congress of Obstetricians and Gynecologists, ACOG Education Pamphlet AP054—Genital Herpes, 2008.
9. Jerry Kennard, "Stigma Revisited," Health Central, December 18, 2008. www.healthcentral.com.

What Is Herpes?

10. John Leo, "The New Scarlet Letter," Time, August 2, 1982. www.time.com.
11. Charles Ebel and Anna Wald, Managing Herpes: Living and Loving with HSV, p. 10. Research Triangle Park, NC: American Social Health Association, 2007.
12. Terri Warren, The Good News About the Bad News: Herpes; Everything You Need to Know. Oakland, CA: New Harbinger, 2009, p. 20.
13. Gayla Baer McCord, "Defining the Differences in Types of HSV," Herpes Online, 2009. www.herpesonline.org.
14. Daniel Ravel, "Oral Herpes and Cold Sores in Children," Pediatric Dental Health, January 25, 2004. http://dentalresource.org.
15. Ebel and Wald, Managing Herpes, p. 34.
16. California Department of Public Health, Summary Guidelines for the Use of Herpes Simplex Virus (HSV) Type 2 Serologies, May 2003. www.cdph.ca.gov.

What Are the Health Effects of Herpes?

17. Charlotte Raveney, "Important News for Everyone to Consider: Newborn Baby Died in Britain Due to Herpes Simplex Virus-1," Luciole Press Blog, October 27, 2008. http://blog.luciolepress.com.
18. Raveney, "Important News for Everyone to Consider."
19. Ebel and Wald, Managing Herpes, p. 146.
20. Quoted in National Institute of Allergy and Infectious Diseases, "Scientists Learn Why Even Treated Genital Herpes Sores Boost the Risk of HIV Infection," press release, August 2, 2009. www.niaid.nih.gov.
21. Lawrence Corey et al., "The Effects of Herpes Simplex Virus-2 on HIV-1 Acquisition and Transmission: A Review of Two Overlapping Epidemics," JAIDS: Journal of Acquired Immune Deficiency Syndromes, March 30, 2004. www.medscape.com.
22. Timothy Schacker, "The Role of HSV in the Transmission and Progression of HIV," Herpes, vol. 8, no. 2, 2001. www.ihmf.com.
23. National Institute of Neurological Disorders and Stroke, "Meningitis

and Encephalitis Fact Sheet," December 18, 2009. www.ninds.nih.gov.

24. Deborah Pavan Langston, "Herpes Simplex Virus in the Eye," *Digital Journal of Ophthalmology*, 2010. www.djo.harvard.edu.

How Can Herpes Be Treated?

25. Quoted in Fred Hutchinson Cancer Research Center, "Stemming the Spread of STDs," *Center News*, January 8, 2004. www.fhcrc.org.

26. Warren, *The Good News About the Bad News*, p. 85.

27. Christopher Scipio, "Herpes and the DMSO Deception," Herpes Nation, October 20, 2007. www.herpesnation.blogspot.com.

28. Elizabeth Boskey, "Is There Any Evidence That Resolve Herpes Is a Herpes Cure?" About.com, August 10, 2009. www.std.about.com.

29. Elizabeth Boskey, "How You Know That HPV Cure, HIV Cure, or Herpes Cure Is Fake," About.com, February 18, 2010. www.std.about.com.

30. Quoted in Mother Nature, "Genital Herpes," 2010. www.mothernature.com.

31. Jared Hanson, "Natural Treatment for Herpes," 2010. www.jaredhanson.com.

How Can the Spread of Herpes Be Prevented?

32. Angela, "Angela," Yoshi2me, 2009. www.yoshi2me.com.

33. Kevin Fenton, "CDC Study Finds U.S. Herpes Rates Remain High," press release, Centers for Disease Control and Prevention, March 9, 2010. www.cdc.gov.

34. Minnesota Department of Health, "Genital Herpes," November 24, 2009. www.health.state.mn.us.

35. Ruth Westheimer, *Dr. Ruth's Guide to Talking About Herpes*. New York: Grove, 2004, p. 150.

36. Quoted in Anne Harding, "Condoms Offer Partial Protection Against Herpes," Reuters, July 13, 2009. www.reuters.com.

37. Herpes Diagnosis, "How Is Herpes Transmitted to Others?" 2010. www.herpesdiagnosis.com.

38. Quoted in David Cameron, "Topical Treatment Wipes Out Herpes with RNAi," Harvard Science, January 21, 2009. www.harvardscience.harvard.edu.

List of Illustrations

Index

Note: Boldface page numbers refer to illustrations.

Picture Credits

About the Author

Charles Cozic holds a bachelor's degree in journalism from San Diego State University. He is married with two children in San Diego and enjoys children's theater and writing children's books.